"Doctors Only"

Recent Titles in
Contributions in Medical Studies

Compulsory Health Insurance: The Continuing American Debate
Ronald L. Numbers, editor

Disease and Its Control: The Shaping of Modern Thought
Robert P. Hudson

Pain, Pleasure, and American Childbirth: From the Twilight Sleep to the Read
Method, 1914–1960
Margarete Sandelowski

Understanding the Liver: A History
Thomas S. Chen and Peter S. Chen

Caring for the Retarded in America: A History
Peter L. Tyor and Leland V. Bell

A History of Ancient Psychiatry
Giusseppe Roccatagliata

"Hydropathic Highway to Health": Women and Water-Cure in Antebellum
America
Jane B. Donegan

The American Midwife Debate: A Sourcebook on Its Modern Origins
Judy Barrett Litoff

Planning for the Nation's Health: A Study of Twentieth-Century Developments
in the United States
Grace Budrys

Essays of Robert Koch
K. Codell Carter, translator

Photographing Medicine: Images and Power in Britain and America since 1840
Daniel M. Fox and Christopher Lawrence

The Tuberculosis Movement: A Public Health Campaign in the Progressive Era
Michael E. Teller

Families and the Gravely Ill: Roles, Rules, and Rights
Richard Sherlock and C. Mary Dingus

"DOCTORS ONLY"

The Evolving Image
of the American Physician

Richard Malmsheimer

Contributions in Medical Studies,
Number 25

GREENWOOD PRESS
NEW YORK • WESTPORT, CONNECTICUT • LONDON

Library of Congress Cataloging-in-Publication Data

Malmsheimer, Richard.
    "Doctors only" : the evolving image of the American physician /
Richard Malmsheimer.
        p.   cm. — (Contributions in medical studies, ISSN 0886–8220 ;
no. 25)
    Bibliography: p.
    Includes index.
    ISBN 0–313–23465–5 (lib. bdg. : alk. paper)
    1. Physicians—United States—History.   2. Physicians in
television—United States—History.   3. Physicians in literature—
History.   I. Title.   II. Series.
    R690.M294   1988
    610'.973—dc19   88–5685

British Library Cataloguing in Publication Data is available.

Library of Congress Catalog Card Number: 88–5685
ISBN: 0–313–23465–5
ISSN: 0886–8220

First published in 1988

Greenwood Press, Inc.
88 Post Road West, Westport, Connecticut   06881

Printed in the United States of America

∞™

The paper used in this book complies with the
Permanent Paper Standard issued by the National
Information Standards Organization (Z39.48–1984).

10 9 8 7 6 5 4 3 2 1

for my family

Some patients, though conscious
that their condition is perilous, recover
their health simply through their
contentment with the goodness of the
physician.

> Hippocrates

That's what we are—gods. And the thing
that holds us together as a group is our
realization of this. We know how the
public feels about us.

> Morton Thompson, *Not As A Stranger*

It may be that only the doctor can pass
muster as a genuine hero in this decade.

> Robert Alley (1985)

Contents

Acknowledgments

I want to acknowledge and express my gratitude to all of the people who have given me aid and comfort during the time that this project has been underway. Especially, I want to thank Professors Clarke Chambers, Theodor Litman, and Mary Turpie (University of Minnesota) whose advice and encouragement during the early years of the project were invaluable.

Thanks are also due to the University of Minnesota's English Department for allowing me to teach an experimental course, Doctors in Literature, in the spring of 1973, and to the students in that course, who were willing to share their ideas about doctors, their reactions to the literature we read, and their discoveries of obscure medical novels.

Many of the novels discussed here would not have been available without the collections and the aid of the library staffs at the University of Minnesota, San Diego State University, the University of California at San Diego, Dickinson College and The Bosler Library (Carlisle, Pa). The assistance they all provided is greatly appreciated.

Throughout the more recent stages of the project, Professor John C. Burnham (Ohio State University) has truly been the ideal editor. Without his encouragement, sustained enthusiasm, and extraordinary patience, the transformation from manuscript to book would not have occurred. Likewise, the support of the editorial staff of Greenwood Press and their willingness to wait repeatedly through "just one more extension" have given me the space and time needed to finish the job.

When I began this inquiry, my perspective and questions were mostly those of a curious onlooker. More recently, my work in hospital settings has broadened that perspective and clarified those questions. For the opportunity to come closer to an insider's view of both the doctor's and the patient's dilemma, let me also express my gratitude to the nursing and medical staffs of the Carlisle Hospital (Carlisle, Pa.) and of the Chambersburg Hospital (Chambersburg, Pa.). They have helped me to see more clearly and to question more effectively.

Clear sight and better questions were also nurtured by the faculty and students with whom I studied in the Department of Counseling, Shippensburg University (Shippensburg, Pa.). Their dedication to finding the actor's view of human experience helped me to see that questions about human behavior are always better raised from *within* the context of those involved.

Among the most involved in all of this (their coming into the world generated the first of the project's many questions) have been my sons, Matthew and Aaron, who deserve special thanks for having good-naturedly shared me with "the damned book" for far longer than we've all wanted. And lastly, and firstly, to my wife, Lonna, the thanks that cannot be expressed; she was there, and she knew.

"Doctors Only"

1

Introduction: Wanting More, Getting Less

THE IMAGE OF THE OMNIPOTENT DOCTOR

The problems facing the American medical profession have been reported, analyzed, debated, interpreted, chronicled, and reinterpreted with extraordinary vigor during recent decades. Yet there has been surprisingly little recognition that some of the most crucial of these problems stem from an underlying cultural process that is rooted in the nature of professions in general, in the particular nature of the medical profession, and in the creation and perpetuation of an untenable image of the doctor as omnipotent and priestlike, an image held by (and often a problem for) patients and doctors alike. That image, a result of the ways in which people incorporate into their lives patterns of behavior found to be crucial to survival, has contributed to a cultural predisposition to hold the entire medical profession in the kind of awe reserved only for those who fulfill crucial roles in people's lives. Because doctors only are thought to be possessed of the power to heal, to cure, and to save lives, they only, among all the professionals, are so thoroughly idealized. Furthermore, the idealization, because it answers people's most basic needs for security and hope, is both tenaciously held to and highly resistant to change. In short, people in our society hold their doctors in awe far less from choice than from necessity.

Such awe is understandable, considering what it allows. Functionally, the doctor-patient relationship is one in which respect and trust must overcome fear and uncertainty. To distrust one's doctor is to be vulnerable in the most fundamental and undesirable of ways. At the same time, this necessary and functional awe and its outward manifestations in patients' deference and unquestioning acceptance often trap doctors in patterns of behavior that hinder a necessary admission of human fallibility. Unable to admit their own limitations easily and openly, doctors, for all their skill and good intentions, are handicapped in their attempts to bring about needed change. Similarly trapped are people who expect that their real-life doctors, like their idealized ones, will be infallible, and who demand continuous proof of that infallibility. Unable to accept doctors for what most all of them are—fallible people of skill and good intention—the public, in its demands for perfection, exerts pressures that work, finally, to the detriment of all concerned.

The idealized image remains intact in spite of its negative side effects. It could hardly be otherwise, given the psychic need to behave in ways that decrease stress and increase one's sense of security. Patients can scoff knowingly at the exaggerated portrayals of television doctors, they can complain about the endlessly rising cost of health care, they can bemoan the inefficiencies and inequities of a system that no longer seems to provide the kind of health care once thought possible and attainable—but when faced with immediate medical need, people's defenses and critical facades crumble. Face-to-face with the realization that medicine and its immediate agent, the doctor, may be all that they have to rely on, people fall back upon and give new life and strength to the idealized image they might otherwise question. The underlying dynamic is based in need and fear and a desire both to survive and thrive. Given those parameters, what people hope for and expect are hardly amenable to significant change.

THE MAKING OF THE MYTH

How Americans have come to expect perfection from their doctors is a striking example of the power of culturally devised and transmitted myths. Such myths, whatever their particular form or place of origin, are neither intentional lies nor malevolent fabrications. Rather, they are a crucial means by which people—in all places and at all times—explain their world and maintain it. Much like the stories, both accurate and exaggerated, that comprise a family's told-about history, myths give people a way to retain and make sense of experience. For this reason, the ability to make myths is central to people's lives.*

The genesis and evolution of one such myth-making phenomenon are evident in the myriad portrayals of doctors in American literature and other media during the past century. From the midnineteenth into the early part

* The complex questions of the genesis of cultural myths, their relationship to the realities of everyday life, and the significance of the disparity between "reality" and "myth" are beyond the scope and intention of this book. Suffice it to say that myths as "structures of meaning" *are* real and functional and necessary in their ability to help people see their worlds more clearly and understand those worlds more fully.

of the twentieth century, as America's health care system grew and made notable improvements in patient care, the idealized image of the doctor grew apace. Ironically, into the midportion of the twentieth century, as the system became more and more overburdened and less effectual, as health care became less accessible and more expensive, there was no similar decline in the character or potency of the image and the myth it supported. If anything, in face of a reality receding further and further from the ideal, the image of the omnipotent and priestlike doctor took on greater strength and purity, and the encompassing mythic structure became more elaborate and carefully refined.

What this inability to reconcile the real with the hoped-for says about people's attitudes and about American culture are questions that can well be answered for the benefit of all concerned. Some of the answers are bound up with the process by which people assimilate, make their own, and act upon the varied images that inform their lives. Because people generate their own needed expectations, it is hardly surprising to find Thursday's actual patient wondering why she is not receiving the kind of care that she remembers from a medical novel read years ago or that she saw depicted on Wednesday afternoon's rerun of "Marcus Welby, M.D." This phenomenon of self-generated expectations may help to explain why there has been a parallel rise both in medical standards and accomplishments *and* in malpractice suits. Rising expectations (fed by the image of the omnipotent and always caring doctor) confronting a less-than-perfect reality can result only in frustration.[1] The individual doctor, aware that such frustration and consequent distrust are inimical both to providing good medical care and to maintaining professional status, is forced to reassert the very image that asks for more than any person can provide. If America's doctors are resistant to any substantial change in the public's conception of their identity and role, one of the prime reasons is the fact that they are rarely allowed to admit their humanity and, hence, their fallibility.

THE NEED TO KNOW

The responsibility for this untenable situation must be shared by doctors and patients alike. Instead of holding tenaciously to an unrealistic image of the doctor as priestly magician, patients would do well to let doctors be people. Likewise, the fondly remembered image of the family physician, always available and all-caring, needs to be seen for what it really is—a benign and distorted anachronism in an increasingly complex world. Similarly, doctors both individually and as organized professionals would be better served if they could see the realities before them, adapt to those realities, and yield more gracefully to change. Doctors, then, as well as their patients and their colleagues in training, need to find some way to understand the yearning that they all share for the actualization of an image whose potency and distortions obstruct the very healing to which all are committed.

To begin to understand the origins and evolution of the distorted and highly evocative image of the American doctor, it is necessary to approach that image from a variety of perspectives. Each of these angles of vision (sociology, history, communications theory, literature, popular culture) is a means to an end. None viewed separately is the central concern of this exploration; that concern—the genesis, transmission, and use of the behaviorial products of cultural forms—is evident only in the interaction of these multiple perspectives.

Each of these perspectives, though important in and of itself, provides only one portion of the whole picture. Like the painting composed of multiple layers of pigment, each layer discrete yet also an integral part of the whole, this study relies on the interaction of its component parts. Each of the following chapters, then, needs to be seen in interrelationship to each and to all of the others.

Chapter 2 considers the nature of the professions in general and moves to a more detailed view of the peculiar tensions inherent in the medical world. These tensions, rooted in the conflict between selflessness and self-interest, make for particular problems in the management of the crucial doctor-patient relationship. It is this relationship, in both its theoretical and actual phases, that provides the study's underlying link between seemingly disparate materials. Medical training and role socialization are viewed in terms of their impact on the doctor-patient relationship and on the expectations they engender for all involved.

Moving from a sociological to an historical perspective, Chapter 3 highlights the evolution of the medical profession in America in order to show the actual backdrop against which the medical idealization was established. The focal point of this historical overview is again the doctor-patient relationship, and especially the changes wrought on it by changes within the profession. The disparity between what people expected of their doctors and what they actually got as the whole health care system changed led, invariably, to a sense of frustration generated by unchanging expectations that were more and more often violated by changing circumstances.

The genesis of those needed expectations and how they are affected by cultural forms provide the focus for Chapter 4. There the particular questions regarding the effect of any given communication are placed within the larger context of cultural transmission and reality maintenance in an attempt to devise a way to see the impact, over time, of particular cultural products.

Those products—in this particular instance literature and television shows, two of the most accessible media—are examined in Chapters 5 through 8 in order to demonstrate the materials through which Americans have come to perceive and articulate their idealized image of the doctor. That idealization has become a predictable literary type because of its ability to continue to satisfy readers' wants and needs and to feed their heightened and unrealistic expectations. Those expectations are catered to in an even more calculated manner by television's versions of the mythic ideal. Available to a mass audience, these present a wished-for distortion of reality that is the logical outcome of the ideal that has been evolving for more than a century.

In the course of that time, then, the idealized doctor has become a familiar and expected cultural form. For good or ill, the mythic contours of the benevolent, always caring, all-powerful, often priestlike ideal are woven tightly into the fabric of people's everyday lives. To see the pervasiveness of the ideal and to understand the tenacity of its hold on people's imaginations are necessary preconditions for understanding and dealing with its consequences. The needed understanding of those consequences comes more readily with the clarity of vision provided by the interlocking frameworks of communications theory, history, and sociology. An understanding of the whole, then, necessarily begins with a sequential understanding of its several parts.

2

Training for Frustration: The Sociological Perspective

PROFESSIONS IN GENERAL

What people come to expect from the professionals who serve them is the result of complex factors operating both directly and indirectly on client and professional alike. None of these factors can be fully understood in isolation, and the nature of their interaction requires a discrete and sequential examination of what is, in operation, a total and spontaneous process. To understand, it is necessary to unravel; to apprehend the figure in the carpet, it is necessary first to look at the several threads that go to make up its design. And to do this, to understand these factors, it is necessary to start with a question of definition.

Although early attempts at establishing a working definition of "profession" often resulted in confusion and apparent contradiction,[1] the sociology of the professions provides adequate guidelines in this regard. In broad terms, "a profession is an occupation which has achieved a special level of prestige in society."[2] More specifically, "it is a type of higher-grade, non-manual occupation, with both subjectively and objectively recognized occupational status, possessing a well-defined area of study or concern and providing a definite service, after advanced training and education."[3] Whereas the several professions share numerous characteristics, they are fundamentally defined (and differentiated from other occupations) by the particular kind of knowledge that informs and engenders them. Quite simply, those who comprise the professions know more about the most crucial aspects of people's lives: "Professionals *profess*. They profess to know better than others the nature of certain matters, and to know better than their clients what ails them or their affairs."[4] It is, then, "the application of an intellectual technique to the ordinary business of life, acquired as the result of prolonged and specialized training [which] is the chief distinguishing characteristic of the profesions."[5]

Whereas the professions depend for their very existence on this shared trait of dealing intellectually with the most important areas of human concern, they also share other essential features. Even though, as Bernard Barber points out, "there is no absolute differentiation between professional and other kinds of occupational behavior, but only relative differences with respect to certain attributes common to all occupational behavior,"[6] it is still possible to categorize the behavior of professionals. Barber's own description is useful:

> Professional behavior may be defined in terms of four essential attributes: a high degree of generalized and systematic knowledge; primary orientation to the community interest rather than to individual self-interest; a high degree of self-control of behavior through codes of ethics internalized in the process of work socialization and through voluntary associations organized and operated by the work specialists themselves; and a system of rewards (monetary and honorary) that is primarily a set of symbols of work achievement and thus ends in themselves, not means to some end of individual self-interest.[7]

Barber's mention of a "system of rewards" points to the second characteristic that is essential to the very existence of a profession, that is, the recognition and esteem of the people whom the profession serves. Without this recognition and positive response on the part of the public, no occupation could realize its claim to professional status. The very fact that "all studies show that the public ranks the professions at the top of the occupational prestige hierarchy,"[8] emphasizes the crucial nature of societal approval. Just as a profession depends for its genesis and growth on the particular nature of its intellectual activity, so does it depend for its continued vitality on the esteem granted to it by the public it serves. Without recognition and consequent esteem, no occupation, regardless of its nature and activity, could come to be accepted as a profession.[9]

Professions, then, are defined not only by what their members do but also by how society responds to that activity. Society, however, does not grant its esteem absolutely; at all times, it reserves the right to withdraw that esteem from its doctors, lawyers, clergy, teachers, and such. The reason for society's reservations, the reason for its ambivalence toward the professions is deceptively simple: people are afraid of the expertise that professionals exercise on their behalf. Fundamental as it is, this fear is a potential threat to the prestige and influence of any profession. In *Professional Lives in America*, Daniel H. Calhoun studied physicians, lawyers, and the clergy during the years 1750–1850 and found that an underlying factor in people's ambivalence toward those groups was "an old popular feeling that the learned man, the professional, had found access to some special, genuine knowledge that made him at once useful and dangerous to the rest of humanity."[10] What professionals know is crucial to the lives of those they serve, but that very knowledge often elicits the public's fear that those who know so much may use what they know in ways dangerous to the community at large. Thus the very knowledge and consequent expertise that engender society's esteem also generate its latent fear and mistrust.

This paradox lies at the heart of the relationship between professionals and their public, and it contributes to the second major cause of people's ambivalence toward the professionals who touch their lives. Professional expertise and excellence are seen as explicitly useful while still implicitly dangerous; they are also seen as the means by which the professions are set apart from the larger society. That this setting apart is inevitable and at times necessary does not negate the fact that it also leads the public to fear that expertise, excellence, and control over significant areas of people's lives may, in time, threaten social equality. As Calhoun points out, "Talk about 'excellence' titillates Americans. It also disturbs them, because it seems to endanger equality in a society that has all the resources and the complexity to nurture great inequality.[11] Although Calhoun speaks of a particular American context, the tension he describes between a society's need for professional excellence and its fear of an aristocracy of talent and power arises inevitably from the contradictions that inhere in all professions.[12]

These contradictions arise from the two factors already noted as essential to the very existence of any profession—its own intellectual endeavor and its need for the larger society's esteem. Because a profession's "generalized and systematic knowledge provides powerful control over nature and society, it is important to society that such knowledge be used primarily in the community interest."[13] Unless the community's interests are served in a selfless way, that community will come to limit the esteem without which a profession ceases to be recognized; in fact, ceases to exist. Yet this very demand for selflessness is in perpetual conflict with certain demands of self-interest, demands that also arise from the necessary activities of any profession.

To understand why the professions are continuously forced to balance the demands of selflessness and self-interest, it is helpful to look more closely at some of the activities characteristic of any profession.[14] Once established and recognized as such by the public, a profession must see to its own vitality and growth; it must choose, train, and certify potential members. In doing this, it must reconcile the conflict between society's need for an adequate number of professionals and the profession's need to insure the quality of its members and to minimize excessive competition within its ranks. To achieve balance here, the profession must limit access enough for its own needs, yet not so much that it disregards the needs of society. Of equal importance are the profession's continuous efforts to further the study of its own field and to disseminate new information widely and rapidly. While doing all of these things, the profession must also articulate, both for its members and for the larger public, its standards of conduct, and it must see to it that these standards are upheld. Less altruistically, but with equal concern, a profession must be protective of and work to raise its members' status as well as protect its members' interests. This latter concern often leads a profession into intermittent activity as an interest or pressure group, working (or so it would claim) for both its own and society's benefit. Also in its own interest, a profession tends to encourage cooperation as well as social activity among its members, and it concerns itself with its members' economic security.[15]

All of these activities are necessary if a profession is to maintain its vitality and benefit its own members as well as the larger society. These tasks, complex and difficult as they are, have historically been facilitated by the formation of an association or professional organization.[16] Because such an organization can provide aid in carrying out these numerous activities, it becomes an integral part of the profession itself. Yet, as wide-ranging as the scope of its activities may become, the initial impetus for the formation of a professional organization stems from the profession's concern with the state of its own capabilities and with the nature of the public's response to those capabilities. In all stages of a profession's development, its members realize that they must work continually to improve the quality and effectiveness of their endeavors in order to profit themselves and society. The selfless concern with service to others merges here with the self-interested concern with maintaining and profiting from society's needs and approbation. In the mixture of these concerns, it is possible to find the seeds of people's ambivalence toward the professions on which they rely. Knowing how much self-interest influences their own behavior, people rarely free themselves from the suspicion that professionals whom they think should act selflessly are apt, from time to time, to act also on the basis of their self-interest. It is this ambivalence of the served, arising from the twin forces of the server's selflessness and self-interest, that must be understood by professionals if they are to cope with the attitudes and responses they will encounter in their work.

Training its members, then, to cope with this and the other complexities of the professional world they will enter is a crucial task for all professions. In order to insure competence and the continuity necessary for its successful functioning, a profession must attract, recruit, and train its own. In the course of the advanced training and role socialization that occur during professionalization, the neophyte undergoes a complex and difficult rite of passage and emerges a qualified though fledgling professional. Just as other rites of passage can reveal much about the societies of which they are a part, so can the complex rite of professionalization tell much about the society that depends on it.[17]

The process of professionalization is comprised of several elements, each of which must be actualized if the whole process is to achieve its intended goal. Of primary importance is the transmission "of the generalized and systematic knowledge that is the basis of professional performance." Allied to this function is the equally crucial one of fostering "new and better knowledge on which professional practice can be based."[18] The third phase of professionalization, as crucial as those involved with the transmission and improvement of knowledge and expertise, has to do with the ethical socialization of the profession's members-in-training. In this phase, the neophyte comes to learn not only the field, but also how best to utilize that knowledge. What is learned is how to *be* a member of the chosen profession.

Just as the work and concerns of a profession are aided by the formation of professional organizations, so are the vital activities of recruitment and role socialization carried on within the course of professional education. It is during this complex process that "the outlook and values, as well as the skills and knowledge of practitioners are first shaped by the profession"[19] they have chosen. It is this shaping of the total field of a professional's world that allows for a resolution of (or at least an uneasy truce with) the internal contradictions of that world and a balancing of the opposing forces of selflessness and self-interest. Once capable of such resolution or truce, the professional has a chance to understand and deal with the ambivalence of a public that both needs *and* distrusts professional expertise.

The process that generates and controls such expertise is complex and variable across time and the several professions, yet it is also, at root, relatively stable with its basic contours remaining functionally—and necessarily—similar. Thus the following description of medical professionalization, although a generalized construct, is true to the spirit and intention of the process that inducts and initiates women and men into the "correct" ways of being that the profession requires. To know these ways of being is to know medical culture; it is also to begin to know some of the major constraints—both positive and negative—faced directly by doctors and indirectly by their patients as all of them grapple with the implications of the tension between trust and skepticism.

THE DOCTORS' DILEMMA

Whereas all professions are characterized by the tension between selflessness and self-interest, and whereas they must all contend to varying degrees with the public's ambivalence, "perhaps in no other area are the internal contradictions inherent in the concept of 'professionalism' so acute as in the field of medicine."[20] Because it deals with the most crucial of people's concerns, with life and its preservation, medicine touches people's most profound hopes and can elicit their most extreme fears. When satisfied with their doctors, people are lavish with their praise; when dissatisfied, they are equally lavish with their scorn. Speaking of the public's response to critics of the medical profession, Oliver Garceau in 1961 pointed out a tendency that, if anything, has intensified in the intervening years:

> To the extent that professionalism finds a response in public opinion, to that very degree the reaction of a disillusioned public will be only the more violent. People resent having their faiths exposed; they take vengeance on their betrayers. The enemy need only show that doctors are in fact not much better than the rest of a fallible race—which is undoubtedly true—and the group immediately appears grossly villainous.[21]

Whether perceiving its public image as villainous or merely less satisfactory than a demanding public desires, the profession was and is faced with the need to devise ways to allow its members to resolve for themselves, and for their patients, the tensions and contradictions within the profession. Unless these can be incorporated within the continuing work of the profession, the needs of doctors and patients alike will remain unfulfilled. The history of medicine in America, then, can be seen in terms of ever-growing expertise and competence attempting to overcome the effects of the internal contradictions within the profession. As the profession could do more for its public, that public could, increasingly, allay its fears and ambivalence. As long as there seemed to be a close congruence between the hoped-for and the achieved, all was well. To maintain such a congruence, the profession has had to try to train its members to know and deal with the complex world of their work, which demands both expertise and the ability to function well and with ease in the face of the ambiguity generated by the profession's own inner tensions.

To see how these several difficulties are handled by both the medical profession and by individual doctors, it is helpful to see what happens during the years of medical training. It is via the role socialization that occurs during these years that the medical profession molds the student into the professional practitioner. What happens in these years is similar to what happens during the years that any profession sets aside to train its own. This general process, however, takes on a particular coloration in terms of medical training, a coloration that stems from and illuminates the unique nature of the profession.

Writing some three decades ago, Samuel W. Bloom aptly called medical training a "probationary ordeal,"[22] one "which inculcates the requisite technical skills sometimes, and the necessary social attitudes and behavior patterns always."[23] Medical training is an ordeal largely because of the problem of excess; there is simply too much to learn in the period of time set aside to prepare a doctor to enter practice. Although medical school is only the beginning of a life-long process of learning, it is the only time that the medical student has to learn under supervision all that must be known to begin professional life. The medical school decides what is to be taught and how, but it is the student who must determine what to learn and how. The problem is further compounded by the fact that what must be learned is not only academic and technical knowledge, but also attitudes and behavior. All of these things must finally be actualized within the doctor-patient relationship, the successful handling of which is the aim of the whole process.

In their 1961 study, *Boys in White: Student Culture in Medical School*, Howard S. Becker, Blanche Geer, Everett C. Hughes, and Anselm Strauss traced the evolving reactions of medical students to the choices confronting them regarding what they needed to know and how they could best learn it. In spite of changes in medical school curricula in the intervening quarter-plus century, the underlying educational dynamic and consequent problems remain. Although grounded in a particular time and place, the study by Becker and his colleagues demonstrates more general and still extant trends. In spite of changes in medical school admissions policies and curricula, the model of medical socialization that had evolved by mid-century still holds sway. The authors noted that the freshman medical students' characteristic reaction was initially to attempt "to learn it all."[24] This first perspective was based on the belief that even though there was a tremendous amount to learn, all of it had to be learned, since all of it would be needed.

The decision to "learn it all" led inevitably to frustration. The students soon realized that learning everything was impossible, and they modified the initial perspective to one that can be summarized as a belief that "you can't do it all." This modification led them to decide that, although they would still work as hard as ever, they would channel their work in ways that would enable them to concentrate only on what was most important, either to their future medical practice or to the faculty who had to be dealt with in the more immediate context of medical school.[25] Unfortunately, this modification in student attitude still led to frustration and uncertainty, largely because the students were on the whole unable to determine, from their limited vantage point, what was most important for them to know. This difficulty was compounded by the fact that there was no consistent philosophy among faculty members concerning the scope and direction of student efforts. Consequently, the students were again thrown back on their own judgments.

The final modification of the initial perspective took the form of learning "what they want us to know." This choice revealed that, however autonomous students were at times, they were always in the inferior position in a power relationship.[26] The faculty's power to determine the course of the students' progress led students to accept and to act upon what they felt the faculty valued. Deciding to second-guess the faculty, to attempt by whatever means possible short of cheating to learn what is wanted in order to pass exams and "get through school,"[27] was a far different response from the initial decision to "learn it all." Yet it was a decision consistent with the medical student's own movement from an idealistic to a pragmatic approach to the profession and what it entailed. One manifestation of this increasing pragmatism is evident in medical students' decision to specialize. Those decisions were generally not made prior to or even during the first years of training. Rather, as students came to know more about the complexities of medicine and as their perspectives on what to learn shifted, they came to an increased awareness of their own inability to master all that confronted them. It was this awareness of their own limitations that prompted the final decision to specialize.[28]

Once made, the decision was likely to elicit a favorable response from those in positions of power in relation to the student. Kendall and Selvin's study of Cornell's Medical College found evidence to indicate that "the high ranking student at Cornell who maintains an interest in a rotating internship must to some extent go counter to the expectations and advice of the faculty and administration, while the good student who has already developed specialized interests receives support and encouragement."[29] Yet, even with this additional support and with the increased sense of a limited field in which to direct their efforts, students' decisions to specialize could not eliminate once and for all the two-pronged dilemma of excess and uncertainty.

As student-physicians grow into the normative pattern of their profession, they grow into and become better able to deal with the inevitable excess and uncertainty. The layperson's "utopian view of the physician [as master healer] is at variance with the facts. . . . Despite unprecedented scientific advances, the life of the modern physician is still full of uncertainty."[30] Both personal and professional limitations contribute to the reality of what any doctor can do, and the doctor-in-training needs all the aid available to determine where personal limitations and the limitations of the profession begin. Early evidences of and actual preparation for this inherent uncertainty can be seen in the shifting perspectives on what and how to learn. From these perspectives, students fashion their approach to their field as well as the attitudes and demeanor that will characterize their professional role. Throughout the years of formal professionalization, much of medical students' "difficulty in evolving a plan of study lies in the fact that what [they are] really seeking is nothing less than an organized way of learning to think like a doctor."[31]

Learning to think and behave like a doctor becomes, then, the final guideline determining the direction and nature of medical students' efforts, which become more clearly defined and fixed during the clinical years of training. As they come more and more to deal with patients, students place more and more value on those activities that provide them with the opportunity to gain the kind of experience they foresee as useful for their later years of practice. Similarly, students increasingly direct their efforts in attempts to maximize access to situations in which they can exercise responsibility for patients' well-being. Thus, clinical experience and the concomitant opportunity for responsibility take precedence over book learning.[32] Medical students are most fully able to perceive themselves as the doctors they will become when they deal with patients and are responsible for their well-being. The general tendency for individuals to live up to the role expectations of those with whom they are interacting, and to perceive themselves in accordance with those expectations,[33] facilitates the crucial development of a professional self-image, which evolves from the neophyte's ability to actualize in practice those things learned first only in theory. Clearly then, "it is vis-a-vis patients, more than with any other status in their role set, that medical students even as early as the end of their first year of training tend to see themselves as physicians."[34]

THE CRUCIAL RELATIONSHIP

The patient is the most significant "other" in the doctor's professional life. Because this is so, the self-image of the doctor and the evolving self-image of the doctor-in-training are based largely on the responses and expectations of patients. Doctors become not only what they are trained to become but also what they believe their patients expect them to be. Sociologists Peter L. Berger and Thomas Luckmann describe this interactive process succinctly:

> In other words, the self is a reflected entity, reflecting the attitudes first taken by significant others toward it; the individual becomes what he is addressed as by his significant others. This is not a one-sided mechanistic process. It entails a dialectic between identification by others and self-identification, between objectively assigned and subjectively appropriated identity.[35]

The dialectical nature of this process of self-identification explains why the doctor-patient relationship comes to play such an important role in the professionalization of the medical student. In order to satisfy the need for self-confidence, the student must come to internalize and act upon repeated positive reflections of demonstrated competence. Only when this has been done is it possible to attain a perception of oneself "as a capable physician— a perception which is not merely a reflection of judgments made by the faculty in the form of grades."[36] Distinct from those faculty judgments, and of greater importance as medical students come nearer to completing their training, are the daily judgments and responses of patients. Just as a profession can be what it claims to be only when those it serves recognize and reward that claim, so can individual doctors be what they believe themselves to be only when their patients respond to them in a manner that objectifies and validates their own self-perceptions.

Whereas it may appear simple-minded to assert that without patients there would be no doctors, the very simplicity of that statement masks a wide range of complexities. The understanding of these complexities is crucial to a full understanding of both the process of role socialization involved in medical training and of the problems and complexities of the medical profession itself. In short, to understand the profession and its role in society, one must understand the single most crucial component of the profession—the doctor-patient relationship.

Patients and their doctors do not exist in a vacuum. All are individuals with their own unique attributes as well as the attributes derived from the social groups that define and give direction to their lives. Because doctors and patients come to each other out of a multifaceted cultural background that has molded their needs and demands, their relationship is a complex and dynamic one.[37] Yet underlying this complexity and tending to stabilize the vagaries of the relationship are certain factors unique to it, factors that spring from the needs, fears, and hopes of people who place their health and lives in the hands of others.

The most vital component of the doctor-patient relationship is the trust that patients place in their doctors. In need of expertise that is not fully understood, aware that they are in an inferior position in a power relationship, and desirous of results that may not be forthcoming, patients for their own psychic well-being must be able to trust in the ability and self-lessness of their chosen healers. The healers, in order to maintain the trust that they know full well is vital to their own and their patients' well-being, must mask their own uncertainties and limitations behind a guise of competence and confidence. "When the doctor demonstrates his skill by his determination and decisiveness, the patient is usually grateful for such real reassurance; then he is sure he is in capable, trustworthy hands. There is much wisdom in the old medical dictum that 'in any contact between doctor and patient there is room only for one anxious person—the patient.' "[38]

Just as trust within the relationship is crucial to the individual patient and to the individual doctor, so is the generalized aura of trust important to the profession as a whole. Since patients have ready access to few objective criteria by which to judge physicians' competence, trust comes to serve as the means by which anxiety is allayed and ambivalence is laid to rest. Consequently, the profession, balancing continuously the needs of selflessness and self-interest and always in need of society's approbation and esteem, is able to maintain its prestige and power largely on the basis of the public's generalized response, which springs from the trust that underlies the individual doctor-patient relationship.

At the same time that patients and their physicians rely on the cohesive power of trust, that very trust is continually threatened by the most fundamental component of the doctor-patient relationship, the inescapable fact that the patient *needs* medical care.

Medical responsibility, while for most people a good thing, is for the person in whose behalf it is exercised a bad thing in the sense that it could not be exercised at all if it were not for his [or her] own troubles. The doctor can be most fully a doctor only when others have trouble. Perhaps this ambiguity in the moral aura of the value [of medical responsibility] has something to do with the public's ambivalence toward doctors.[39]

Because the public's ambivalence continually threatens to undermine the trust without which the profession could not function and thrive, the individual practitioners, aware of the precarious balance of these conflicting forces, must do all they can to quell their patients' doubts and fears. "The doctor, aware that an essential requisite of successful treatment is to acquire and retain the confidence of his [or her] patient, and believing that the patient is incapable of appreciating the situation of the art of medicine, tends to a pompous assumption of knowledge and authority . . . [and projects] an atmosphere of miracle and mystery."[40]

Whether one describes the doctor's pose as one of necessary determination and decisiveness or as one of pompously assumed knowledge and authority depends more on one's own point of view than on observable fact. Yet, whatever its particular contours and however they are described, the pose itself is one that grows largely in response to the needs and demands of patients. That these demands are often excessive is understandable, given the crucial nature of the doctor's service and the nature of the patient's response to it. Regardless of the actual severity of the given condition and in spite of the realization that even the best of doctors can only do so much, the patient is still susceptible to "ir- and non-rational beliefs and practices."[41] Patients' potential irrationality is further intensified by their deep-seated ambivalence toward the expertise being exercised in their behalf. Unable to accept and resolve this ambivalence and the uncertainties it engenders, patients come to expect and to demand far more than the realities of medicine can provide.

The complex question of the genesis, growth, and effect of such expectations is the focus of the following chapters. Suffice it here to say that patient's expectations and the demands, both implicit and explicit, that spring from those expectations play a crucial and often questionable role in the doctor-patient relationship. Furthermore, the long-range effects of these expectations tend to force the whole profession to assume a pose of certitude and unqualified competence that is contrary to the actual state of affairs and inimical to open and honest dealings between the profession and its public. "The physician is not, by virtue of his modern role, a generalized 'wise man' or sage—though there is considerable folklore to that effect— but a specialist whose superiority to his fellows is confined to the specific sphere of his technical training and expertise."[42]

When the profession is forced, by the expectations and demands of its public, to transcend the particular sphere of its expertise, it is placed in a position that is precarious and fraught with potential dangers, the most wide-reaching of which is the ever-increasing disparity between the realities of medical practice and the perception, understanding, and distortions of those realities by the general public. Patients who expect their doctors to provide more than is possible and doctors who appear to promise more than they can provide are both self-deceived and deceiving. In their mutually needed deceptions are contained the seeds not only of their own discontent but also of a more pervasive and debilitating public disenchantment with the actual and beneficial fruits of medical expertise.[43]

3

Disillusionment and Discontent: The Historical Dimension

THE PREPROFESSIONAL PERIOD: 1650–1850

Historical and social forces and the cultural artifacts arising from them have produced a situation in which the expectations of the American public have been raised far beyond the level at which they can be satisfied by the medical profession. To see how this is so, it is helpful to view the doctor-patient relationship as it has evolved within the context of the growth and change of the medical profession in America. To chart that growth in full, to present even a condensed version of medicine in America, is not the intention of this work. However, a look at the highlights of that process is useful in clarifying the evolution of the doctor-patient relationship.[1] It is that relationship and its changes over time that will provide the focal point of the historical considerations that follow. Seeing the forces that have affected the doctor-patient relationship through three centuries lays the groundwork for seeing how Americans have produced an ongoing myth of invincible and arcane medical expertise, a myth that has been and continues to be a problem for those who partake of it.

Speaking of medicine in America in the years from 1620 to 1820, the medical historian Richard Harrison Shryock notes that it provided little more than "1.) moral and psychosomatic values, 2.) minor amelioration . . . , 3.) the handling of structural emergencies, and 4.) occasional checks to contagion."[2] Still based on a medieval humoral pathology, that defined medical care in terms of the maintenance of particular bodily systems rather than in terms of the treatment of specific disease entities,[3] medical thought and the practice dependent on it could offer little of real value to those it served. Compounding the difficulty in the American colonies was the fact that there was little formal training among those who practiced medicine. Since few British physicians had emigrated, virtually anyone who behaved like a general practitioner was accepted as such.[4] In the century before the American Revolution, medicine was largely in the hands of lay-practitioners who took to doctoring as a sideline.

Among these lay-practitioners was a substantial number of women, who, because of their abilities and society's needs, were encouraged to provide whatever care they could. In the half-century preceding the Revolution, however, women were less and less accepted as substitutes for the more normative medical men.[5] With this decline in the number of medical women, most of the lay-practitioners in the decades prior to the Revolution were educated men—planters, magistrates, clergy—with no formal medical training. On the eve of the American Revolution there were upward of 3,500 established practitioners serving a colonial population of two million. Of these, not more than 400 had received any formal training. Of the 400, only about half (or 5 percent of the total number of practitioners) held any sort of degree;[6] the rest had been trained by apprenticeship. Given this paucity of trained practitioners, it is not surprising that there were few attempts to impose standards via licensing controls. The colonists, in need of the care available, as minimal as that was, were not inclined to limit the activities of their lay healers. Although apt to prefer educated physicians, the colonists took what they could get. Also, because of the great disparity between public need and the available number of formally trained doctors, there was, through the early decades of the eighteenth century, little conflict between the trained and the untrained doctors in the colonies.[7]

During the years that medical care was in the hands of lay-practitioners, there was for all practical purposes no medical science in the colonies.[8] The more immediate and pressing demands of minimal patient care were simply not compatible with the conditions necessary for a science of medicine. A further effect of this practical orientation can be seen in the dearth of medical writing prior to the 1730s; what little existed was generally directed to the needs and requirements of a popular audience.[9] The foremost exception to the nonscientific and necessarily practical orientation of medicine in the colonial years was the success achieved in 1721 by the Reverend Cotton Mather and the apprentice-trained Dr. Zabdiel Boylston in their attempts to innoculate against smallpox in Boston. Violently opposed by the public and by other physicians, Mather and Boylston did succeed in averting an epidemic. Their achievement was unparalleled in American medicine until the middle of the nineteenth century.[10]

Had Boylston and Mather's work been more widely known and accepted, it is still unlikely that it would have been able to encourage even the beginnings of anything approaching a distinctly American medicine. The first half of the eighteenth century saw American physicians increasingly influenced by continental theory and practice. Not only were they ever more aware of developments overseas, but also in the years following 1730 they traveled in increasing numbers to Leyden in the Netherlands, to Edinburgh and London for training as yet unavailable in the colonies. With few opportunities for formal training at home and with even less public support for theoretical work, it is understandable that there were no notable discoveries made by American doctors in either basic or applied science during the eighteenth century.

Although there was no medical science as such in America during the colonial period, there were, in the middle decades of the eighteenth century, the beginnings of progress in terms of professional and institutional developments.[11] In 1751, the Pennsylvania Hospital, the first hospital in the modern sense of the word, was established in Philadelphia, and by 1760 that city was becoming the chief American medical center. The College of Philadelphia's medical school was founded in 1765, and three years later, King's College (now Columbia University) opened its medical school, as did Harvard College in 1783. Yet, even though the opportunities for formal training both in America and abroad were increasing, the actual practice of medicine could make little headway until medical science freed itself from its medieval inheritance of a nonempirical humoral pathology. The institutions needed for the transmission of medical knowledge were being established. What they lacked and had to wait for until the beginning of the nineteenth century was a body of medical knowledge attainable only when rational speculation was replaced by intelligent and effective empiricism.

The latter half of the eighteenth century witnessed, first in Europe and then in America, a growing distrust of speculation and a consequent rise in the respect accorded empirical study. The gradual decline of extravagent theories was coupled with a growing realization of the need to correlate clinical and pathological findings in order to be able to begin to systematize, classify, and eventually disseminate new medical knowledge. A growing faith in the capabilities of science was nurtured by the recognition that empiricism, previously condemned, could yield results of a tangible and increasingly significant nature. Throughout these years, doctrine and dogma from the past were continually questioned and discarded to make way for a new medical science. Once freed from the encumbrances of its past, medicine could begin to move into its modern phase.[12]

As doctors in America awaited the developments that would eventually provide them with a coherent and systematic body of knowledge, they began to experience stirrings of discontent within their ranks. As more of them received formal training, both at home and abroad, it became possible for the first time to differentiate between varying degrees of competence. Those who perceived themselves as more competent began to feel threatened by the proliferation of untrained practitioners, and they were anxious to thin the ranks of the untrained. The earlier rapport between learned and unlearned doctors diminished in the face of growing competition and a growing public demand for better care. Yet the earliest moves on the part of trained practitioners to establish licensing restrictions were rebuffed by the public, who viewed such activities as the work of incipient monopolists trying to limit medical care for their own benefit.[13]

Even though concern with licensing grew throughout the latter half of the eighteenth century, there was no possible way to actualize this concern effectively while the public's need for care of any sort so greatly exceeded the ability of even minimally qualified doctors to satisfy that need. Thus, even though New York and New Jersey had set up the mechanisms for state licensure before the Revolution and even though most other states followed suit by 1810, there were by 1820 still too few trained doctors to let licensure become effective. Similarly, even though by 1815 nearly all the states possessed medical societies, these societies could do little to control physicians' behavior.

In short, there were virtually no restraints on medical practitioners, and by the beginning of the nineteenth century "competition in practice was a free for all."[14] This scramble for patients tended, continually, to threaten the precarious balance that was slowly being established between public need and medical competence. Among better trained doctors who viewed themselves as America's medical elite, there was, by 1820, a growing optimism. In their eyes medical schools and hospitals of quality were being established and a guild of trained and identifiable doctors was growing larger.[15] Further bolstering this optimism was the doctors' belief that health conditions had improved slightly in the last half of the eighteenth century. Whether such a belief was statistically verifiable did not matter to those who held it. What did matter was that it allowed doctors to view their work as increasingly effective and worthy of public approbation.

Patients, however, neither shared in the belief of improved care nor did they grant their esteem unreservedly. Death rates were still high, and many of the courses of treatment prescribed, especially excessive bleeding and the use of large doses of purgatives, left patients so treated wondering whether their initial illness might not have been preferable to its supposed cure. One response to the prevalence of such "heroic practices" was growing public reliance on a proliferation of medical sectarians who promised that cures could be effected by far milder means. Homeopathic physicians, who believed that minute doses of drugs causing certain symptoms were able to cure diseases exhibiting those same symptoms, competed for favor with Thomsonians who based their cures on the use of vegetable remedies. The popularity of these and other medical sectarians and cultists testified to the uncertain state of public trust in more formally trained "regular" physicians.

In spite of the elite's claims to competence and better judgment, the public responded practically by rewarding those physicians who *seemed* to achieve results regardless of their training and methods. It was less the often cited egalitarianism of Jacksonian democracy than a desire for tangible results that allowed all forms of medicine to have an equal chance of acceptance in the early decades of the nineteenth century. With few objective criteria upon which to base their choice of a physician, Americans, believing themselves capable of choosing wisely, were as likely to consult a quack as they were to choose a trained doctor.[16]

Further complicating the situation was the public's tendency to view disease as an inevitable state of affairs. Well into the nineteenth century, "Americans continued to view illness as a misfortune to meet *after* it occurred. Medical men were expected to restore health rather than preserve it."[17] This underlying belief in disease as part of the natural order of things led to continued indifference to all attempts to institute public health measures. It also led to and reinforced patients' tendencies to choose doctors who promised fast and easy cures while disregarding the more important long-range goals of preventive medicine.

Not even the cholera epidemics of the nineteenth century were able to change the public's belief that disease was inevitable and the result of a sinful life. Cholera "could not alter existing patterns of thought. It reinforced convictions; it could not change them."[18] One of the convictions reinforced by the epidemics was the belief that regular practitioners were virtually powerless to deal with the disease. The public's skepticism did not go unnoticed by doctors already struggling against the burdens of geographical and intellectual isolation, poor pay, and little training. In conjunction with these other liabilities, the epidemics threatened credibility and prestige. Worse still, they called into question doctors' own confidence and world view.[19]

Doctors were unable to meet this challenge in 1832, and the epidemic "shook an already insecure public confidence."[20] The epidemic of 1849 further demonstrated the medical community's inability to achieve tangible results and further undermined public trust and physicians' status. By the time of the epidemic of 1866, even though medical science was advancing, few practical results were evident; consequently, physicians' status and the public's belief in what they could do were not appreciably different from what they had been two decades earlier.[21]

Dramatic and devastating as it was, however, cholera was not the sole or even primary cause of the decline of doctors' tenuously held status and of the deterioration of the doctor-patient relationship during the first three-quarters of the nineteenth century. The epidemics merely accentuated underlying forces already at work. One such force that undermined the quality of medical care and, consequently, lowered the public's esteem was the proliferation of medical schools, which led in a short time to a lowering of standards and to an objective decline in doctors' competence. Initially, the establishment of new schools was a direct response to the nation's need for more doctors, a need occasioned by a growing native population, increased immigration, and westward migration. Between 1810 and 1840, twenty-six new schools were founded; between 1846 and 1876, forty-seven more came into existence; and between 1873 and 1890, 114 others opened their doors.[22] As the number of medical schools grew, the standards of many of them declined. In order to attract and hold the number of students needed to maintain their financial stability, and, in the case of the growing number of proprietary schools, to turn a profit from high enrollments, "most schools admitted youths without higher education and with uncertain secondary school backgrounds."[23]

As the quality of medical students declined, so did the quality of the education they received. Whereas Shryock notes in comparatively neutral fashion that the quality of medical education declined in the first half of the nineteenth century, "in an absolute sense,"[24] Joseph F. Kett provides a more striking description of this decline in *The Formation of the American Medical Profession* as he cites the thesis of Andrew Boardman, a graduate of the Geneva (New York) Medical College, who describes his own mediocre preparation:

> Boardman cited the teaching of chemistry by a Doctor of Divinity and the absence of physiology lectures as typical of conditions. The "Western Hospital," advertised as providing adequate clinical facilities, had turned out to be the second floor of a shoe store. The anatomy class had been provided with only one cadaver for the entire course. Geneva's standards were no worse than those of many rural and some urban medical schools. If regular physicians were to answer the sectarian accusation that their ranks were riddled with incompetents, reforms had to be launched.[25]

Although the need for reform came to be recognized more and more fully, the very growth of the medical establishment worked against effective reform measures. Rival medical schools were unwilling to raise their admission standards and slow to improve their training. As more schools turned out more and more nominally "trained" practitioners, competition for patients led regular physicians to assert their own competence with more and more vigor while questioning with equal vigor the ability of many of their peers. Only gradually did they come to see that such quarrels, often aired in public, were damaging the reputations of all doctors.[26] Not until the last quarter of the century were they also able to see that widespread incompetence was an even greater threat to the success of all those who possessed even minimal ability.

Further intensifying medical competition and indicating the decline of public trust in regular physicians was the rise of medical sectarianism, the proliferation of quackery, and the growth of the patent medicine and popular health journal industries.[27] With less and less apparent reason to trust regular, trained doctors, patients in ever-increasing numbers asserted their right to choose from a wide variety of quacks and nostrums. The regulars, unable to guarantee the results their patients wanted, had few means to counter such public desertions. Internal squabbles, the decline of medical training, the actual surplus of doctors with its attendant difficulties, the continual failure of attempts to limit practice only to orthodox physicians— all of these factors led to regular medicine's increasingly weak position. And "last but not least among the handicaps of the regular guild was the limited effectiveness of their own practice."[28] Not until regular medicine could prove itself demonstrably superior to its competition could it expect to gain public trust and support.

At the same time that doctors of all stripes were giving the public ample reason to mistrust them, other forces were at work to heighten the public's cynicism. Expanded publishing facilities coupled with rising literacy gave medicine's critics a growing audience.[29] The same audience that read of physicians' shortcomings also learned of the practical successes in physical science and came to wonder about medicine's failure to contribute to human welfare on anywhere near the same scale. Public mistrust was fed by the growing feeling that medical science and medical practice were falling behind; a question that often came to mind was "where were the *medical* equivalents of the steam engine or the telegraph?"[30] By the middle of the century, public sentiment, even among patients who still believed in their own particular doctor, was unprecedentedly negative, and the effects of that negativism were becoming increasingly visible to the medical establishment: " 'The profession to which we belong,' the first president of the American Medical Association declared [in 1848], 'has become corrupt, and degenerate, to the forfeiture of its social position, and with it, of the homage it formerly received spontaneously and universally.' "[31]

AN EMERGING PROFESSION: 1850—1870

In 1850 doctors in America had no way to lay claim to professional status. Medical science had not yet been able to provide a usable and effective body of generalized and systematic knowledge for doctors to use. Medical education was increasingly unable to maintain, much less raise, standards. Medical practice, beset by excessive competition and growing incompetence, was equally unable to provide consistent results. Doctors, far from being able to police their own ranks in the interest of insuring a minimal level of competence, were continually at odds concerning the questions of internal or external regulation and colleague control. And public esteem, crucial to the very existence and vitality of the profession, was at an all-time low.

Voluntary associations, in the form of county and state medical societies, were unable to improve the situation. Although they did provide members with a forum for airing their grievances, they could do little to influence state legislatures to enact effective controls via new licensing laws, and they could do even less to raise the public's esteem. Yet, with all of their limitations, the medical societies of the 1830s and 1840s did lay the groundwork for the kind of voluntary association that would, within the next fifty years, allow the medical community to control itself and begin to attain its long-sought status as a profession.

An event that occurred at the New York Academy of Medicine in the winter of 1847–48 was indicative of American doctors' growing realization of the need to set their house in order. In two speeches delivered on behalf of the academy, John W. Francis, one of the leaders of New York's medical community, took a public stand against individualism and idiosyncracy among his colleagues. His call for conformity was advanced as an antidote to the competitiveness and factionalism that were splintering the medical community in New York, but his concern was shared by doctors throughout the country. "He spoke to the particular need of New Yorkers and New York physicians; but he also spoke to the needs of all American doctors."[32]

Those needs—conformity, quality, and a broad-based sense of colleagueship and strengthened association—were also the motivating force behind the formation of the American Medical Association (AMA), which grew out of a national convention held in New York City in 1846 and attended by more than one hundred delegates from medical colleges and societies in sixteen states. The 1847 convention, held in Philadelphia, drew 250 representatives from twenty-one states, and at the third meeting, held in Baltimore in 1848, the name American Medical Association was adopted.[33] Just as John Francis had extolled the virtues of conformity as an antidote to deviance and factionalism, so did the newly formed national association exhort its members as well as its nonmember colleagues to police themselves in order to improve medical practice and win the public's esteem. The association maintained that only by restricting entry into the profession as well as by purging incompetents from within their ranks could the country's regular trained doctors overcome their burdens of factionalism, competition, and public distrust.

Yet for all its attempts to control the medical community it claimed to represent, the American Medical Association was able to do little on either the state or national levels in the first decades of its existence. The association's early efforts at self-regulation were foredoomed by what Kett describes as a "fundamental flaw in the idea of voluntary associations."

Voluntary self-regulation is invariably complicated by the contradictory forces of altruism and self-interest. A voluntary association, if it is to succeed in strengthening its members' position in society, must improve the service that its members provide. To do this, it must establish standards, enforce them, and eliminate the less competent. However, this rite of purification runs counter to an association's need for broad-based membership, without which professional accord and conformity are unattainable. Thus the struggling American Medical Association was faced, from its inception, with the

dilemma of how to improve medical practice without alienating and ex-
cluding large numbers of physicians whose participation and support were
crucial to the association's viability.[34] Since the national association drew
its representation from the state associations, which were similarly composed of the representatives from county medical associations, there was
no way for the association as a whole to claim that it was succeeding in
purifying its ranks while member doctors at the local level still adhered to
practices that drew condemnation from the national organization and from
the public.

Further compounding the difficulties that arose from the conflicting demands of purity and rapport was the public's ironic reluctance to accept
the kind of restrictions on doctors that the AMA advocated. In its repeated
calls for a lengthened and improved period of training, the association
showed little appreciation of "the distinctive aspects of either American
medical education or American society."[35] The call to recast American medical education in a European mold disregarded the fact that standards were
high in Europe precisely because there were very few medical schools and
few trained physicians. The bulk of European medical practice was left to
lay-practitioners who were no better qualified than the average graduate of
America's medical colleges. To lengthen the term of medical training and
to restrict entry to medical schools by raising entrance requirements would
have raised standards just as achieving more stringent licensing procedures
would have done. But all of these actions depended on the existence of an
adequate number of competent physicians who could answer the public's
health needs *after* the less competent practitioners had been eliminated. By
the midnineteenth century, most areas of the country could not afford to
do without their less well trained doctors. The choice was rarely between
superior quality and mediocrity, but rather between minimal competence
and nothing at all.[36]

Although when healthy, people feared and mistrusted physicians in general to an unprecedented degree, the individual patient in need of treatment
was unwilling to reject the help, however minimal, of whichever doctor was
available. The public's ambivalence was further intensified by the overall
ineffectiveness of American medicine. Since the visible record of medical
practice of all sorts provided little to distinguish between the self-proclaimed,
competent doctors and their disparaged competitors, there was little public
support for measures that would, *in the public's mind*, serve only to limit
access to needed care while serving to benefit the monopolistic tendencies
of elitist physicians. Until American medicine could demonstrate its effectiveness widely and consistently, there could be little hope of eliciting public
support for any significant attempts to purify and upgrade the medical
community. Similarly, public support for needed medical research was weakened by the general belief that since medical science should function to
provide useful knowledge, there was no reason to assist it when it failed to
achieve that purpose.[37] By the beginning of the Civil War (1861–65), then,

medicine in America had established the institutional structures—hospitals, medical schools, voluntary associations, and such—needed to improve itself and to attain professional status. But not until the potential inherent in those structures could be actualized and brought to bear on the needs of the public, not until the hoped-for was transformed into tangible results would patients be able to grant doctors the esteem necessary for American medicine to become, truly, the profession it had aspired to be for two centuries.

COMING OF AGE: 1870–1920

The last third of the nineteenth century saw American medicine begin to free itself of the twin burdens of provincialism and mediocrity and move toward the start of its modern age. Crucial to this change was the effect of German science and training: "The recovery of medicine in the last decades of the nineteenth century coincided with the rise to leadership of men trained in Germany or subjected to German influence, and with the concomitant introduction of laboratory medicine and training in the basic sciences."[38] Even a brief catalogue of the accomplishments of these decades makes clear why medicine in both Europe and America became, in a relatively short period, a phenomenon to be thought of in new ways. Although many of the most striking accomplishments had been in preparation for years, the singular fact that so much seemed to come to fruition so rapidly gave a skeptical and often hostile public reason to pause and reassess its own judgement of the profession.

Decades of study in parasitology and bacteriology culminated, via the work of French chemist Louis Pasteur and British surgeon Joseph Lister, in the ability to prevent surgical infections. Now able to control infection, surgeons could finally bring their skill to bear on medical problems with increasing effectiveness. In the 1870s Pasteur and German scientist Robert Koch demonstrated that it was possible to isolate specific disease agents, a discovery crucial to further developments in preventive medicine. Complementing advances in preventive medicine was a growing awareness of the value of sanitary reform and other public health measures in reducing sickness and contagion and in maintaining good health. A more dramatic combatant of disease came through advances in structural pathology, which made it possible to determine cellular reaction to specific drugs. Once this determination was possible, a systematic search for remedies against particular diseases could be launched.[39]

Although these crucial developments occurred in Europe, their effects were soon known and put into practice in the United States. As a result, American medicine began to recover from the factionalism and incompetence that undercut and obscured the genuinely good work of the profession's best members. This recovery, most fully embodied in the opening of the Johns Hopkins Medical School in Baltimore in 1893, had been building slowly throughout the latter half of the nineteenth century. The improvements in medical training that were instituted at Johns Hopkins and copied at other of America's better medical schools solidified the growing improvements in medical practice and, consequently, helped to revitalize the profession.[40] In the next decades, advances in surgery, widening applications of endocrinology and nutritional studies, and successes in serum and chemotherapy led to new and more positive attitudes about and within the ranks of America's doctors.[41]

Not only was the medical profession itself revitalized, but the public, increasingly aware of the day-to-day benefits accruing from both medical science and practice, had positive reasons to view its physicians in a new light. Between 1870 and 1920 the major plagues—smallpox, tuberculosis, diptheria, and others—were brought under control for the first time in history.[42] As would be expected, these accomplishments were acknowledged and rewarded. By the turn of the century, the status of physicians had begun to improve noticeably and would rise to unprecedented heights in the next fifty years. As public confidence grew, the individual patient's attitude toward her or his own doctor changed for the better: "The family doctor inspired a feeling of personal confidence, the specialist a sense of warmth."[43] Paralleling the rise of public esteem was an unprecedented rise in the number and amount of financial subsidies—both governmentally and privately funded—granted for medical research. Medicine, finally able to show that it worked, began to reap the rewards bestowed by a public that had long hoped for what its doctors were finally beginning to provide.

DISEQUILIBRIUM AND DISCONTENT: THE YEARS SINCE 1920

The same years that saw the start of American medicine's transformation also witnessed profound changes in the larger society. In the decades following the Civil War, the United States became an urbanized, industrialized, and bureaucratized nation, which relied increasingly on government involvement in people's day-to-day affairs to maintain order and facilitate continuous development. As Robert H. Wiebe points out in *The Search For Order 1877–1920*, a new middle class of aspiring professionals emerged during these years and became the functioning handmaidens of a system of bureaucratic capitalism that relied on those professionals to foster and maintain the continuity, regularity, and rationality essential for the system's growth.[44]

Among these aspiring professionals were the nation's doctors, who, by the turn of the century, had come to see the benefits that they, too, could derive from partaking of the organizational impulse that was sweeping the country. In the 1890s, after four decades of virtually ignoring the American Medical Association, doctors nationwide recognized the advantages to be gained from strengthening their local medical societies and bringing them together under the banner and influence of the nationally based AMA. Between 1900 and 1910, AMA membership grew from 8,400 to 70,000; by 1920, 60 percent of the country's physicians were members. With such greatly enlarged membership and consequently expanded influence, the association moved to limit entry into the profession in an attempt to improve medical education and practice. Similarly, it undertook the task of upgrading the skills of older doctors as well as reorienting and modernizing older and recalcitrant medical schools.[45]

Re-education and reorientation were aided by the Carnegie Foundation for the Advancement of Teaching, which commissioned educator Abraham Flexner to survey America's medical schools. Flexner's observations further strengthened reform efforts that had already been in the works for a full decade. His judicious and compelling *Report* of 1910 was heeded by laypeople and professionals alike, and their response hastened the closing or upgrading of inadequate schools nationwide.[46]

The closing of second-rate medical schools was a victory for the American Medical Association, which had for six decades made intermittent though futile attempts at reforming medical education. Ironically, the victory could not have been won except for the timely intervention of state governments, an intervention that served the profession's immediate purposes but also raised the spectre of external control that was even then and still remains anathema to American medicine. Never before had the profession been so well able to use governmental power to achieve its own ends. Never again would the two forces be able to cooperate so readily for the good of both the profession and the public.

Having begun to come into its own by the beginning of the twentieth century, American medicine was anxious to consolidate its gains and solidify its position. While doing this, the profession fought vigorously to retain its autonomy in the face of the more general trend toward government involvement in all spheres. Unlike the growing corporations, which had come to realize that "social reform" handled correctly could be genuinely conservative[47] and that government intervention could, in fact, aid the growth of a rationalized and bureaucratized corporate state if the "right kind" of regulation were fostered, the medical profession came more and more to contest any interference in its domain.[48] Not only was the profession's response to government intervention into any and all medical affairs increasingly anachronistic as the twentieth century progressed, but the traditional mode of medical practice became less and less able to keep pace with changes in both the profession and the larger society. As medical knowledge expanded and medical technology became increasingly sophisticated, the solo practitioner, the model for the profession, became less and less able to stay abreast of developments. Similarly, as the demand for medical care grew and as the number of doctors engaged in patient care work declined, the health care system, built on the independent activity of the doctor-entrepeneur, became less and less able to fulfill the nation's medical needs.

Further compounding the problem was the fact that the profession chose to define and defend itself primarily in terms of the outdated and overburdened relationship between the single doctor and his or her patient. That relationship was sanctified and used continually as a defense against any form of external control; anything that would damage it was to be resisted at all costs.

In his perceptive study, "The Doctor: Change and Conflict in American Medical Practice," Wayne G. Menke documents the success with which the medical profession resisted "increasing pressures for the revision of the professional conception of the physician's role in American society."[49] The profession's resistance to change was based largely on the fear that its prestige, income, and individual freedom were "threatened by . . . plans for insurance company or government practice" and on the corollary fear that its critics were trying "to regiment medical practice along industrial lines."[50] Fearful of external control, American medicine became, in the words of sociologist Everett C. Hughes, "the avowed enemy of bureaucracy, at least of bureaucracy in medicine when other than physicians have a hand in it."[51]

This antibureaucratic impulse, occurring within the context of a society that was becoming increasingly dependent on bureaucratic development as the means to insure continuity and growth, led the country's doctors to fall back on the evocative power of the doctor-patient relationship as their final defense against change. Menke details well the effects of using this idealized and increasingly overburdened relationship as the means to counter the bureaucratization of medicine. The very patients who had come to believe in and rely on the relationship and rapport they had with a single physician also came more and more to expect (and demand) a higher quality medical care attainable only within an increasingly complex and organized medical system. Doctors were caught in the middle, invariably frustrated in their attempts to reconcile the hoped-for with the real.[52]

When Menke speaks of the kind of medical service that the modern public had been *led to expect,* he points to the underlying cause of the problems arising from the tension between the autonomy embodied in the traditional mode and values of solo practice and the growing therapeutic and organizational imperatives and constraints imposed on medicine in the twentieth century. Regardless of the actual quality of medical care in America, patients who have been led to expect more than any doctor can provide have been increasingly disillusioned during the very decades when medicine has made its most startling advances. Aware of these expectations and of the need to retain their patients' trust, doctors also operate within their own set of expectations. They, too, are unable to free themselves or their patients from those very expectations, which, when frustrated, invariably lead to disillusionment and discontent.

This, then, is the state of disequilibrium through which the doctor-patient relationship has evolved in the past three-quarters of a century. The spiral of expectations has risen at a rate faster than that of medical progress and has been fed invariably by the very progress it continues to outpace. Consequently, patients and doctors, believing in and preferring a form of medical practice less and less able to meet contemporary demands for health care delivery, exist in a relationship that no longer serves the best interests of either group. Yet, as anachronistic and overburdened as it is, that relationship is tenaciously held to by all concerned. Facing the daily realities of medical care while clinging to a remembered—sometimes imagined—past, neither patients nor their doctors have been willing or able to understand, accept, or function within the enormous changes confronting them.

DISILLUSIONMENT

By midcentury, the inability of all concerned to adapt to change had led to the paradox of unprecedented criticism at the very time when the profession was able to manifest unprecedented achievement. One cause of this paradox was the fact, as Shryock pointed out, that "the more people trusted medical aid, the less they could afford it."[53] The techniques and technology that made medical care increasingly effective and trustworthy also made it more and more expensive and less accessible to large numbers of people. Even for those able to cope with the spiraling medical costs, access to primary physician care came to be a problem. The actual shortage of doctors was evident in the severalfold rise in emergency room admissions, in the nation's increased reliance on foreign physicians, and in the fact that fully one-third of all doctors were, by the late 1960s, engaged in work unrelated to patient care.[54] "The National Advisory Commission on Health Manpower in its report to President Johnson cited three leading indicators of crisis [in the availability of doctors]: long delays in obtaining appointments for routine care; hours spent in waiting rooms followed by hurried and impersonal attention; and difficulty in reaching a doctor at night and on weekends, except through hospital emergency rooms."[55] In the two decades since that report, the situation improved little as far as patients could determine, although studies continued to assert that there was an actual and growing surplus of doctors.[56] In spite of what the most carefully established statistics and the projections based on them reported, patients continued to sense that all was not well in the medical world upon which they relied.

For some of the health care system's critics, the problems were accentuated by the fact that Americans did not appear to enjoy the world's best health. Characteristic of these critics was Godfrey Hodgson, who pointed out that "after twenty years of unprecedentedly high expenditure on research, American medicine, far from 'curing everybody,' was unable to prevent public health standards from slipping behind those of many other countries with far smaller resources."[57] The statistics that Hodgson cited—seventeenth in the international league table of infant mortality, fifteenth in female life expectancy, thirteenth in male life expectancy—were pointed to with minor variations year after year by critics anxious to show the "crisis" confronting American medicine.

The actual statistics, however, were then and are now known by only a limited segment of the public. What was and is known, not on a statistical but rather on the highly personal basis of patients' own experiences, is that the health care system seems unable to keep pace with the medical profession's most dramatic achievements. Polio vaccine, antibiotics, kidney transplants, open heart surgery, artificial insemination, genetic engineering—these and other modern "miracles" stand in sharp and disturbing contrast to the everyday problems that patients face in obtaining and paying for more routine care. Thus, although the health care system has in actuality become overburdened and is less than perfect, it is the *perception* of the system's inadequacies that determines the public's response. Regardless of the actual quality of the care available, it is medicine's perceived inadequacies that undermine patient trust and contribute to the deterioration of the doctor-patient relationship.

As the disparity between expectations and perceived reality continues to grow, the disillusionment of those who hope for and demand more than the health care system can provide will only increase. This cycle of frustrated expectations leading to growing disillusionment and criticism is evident in the medical exposé literature of recent decades. Writers of all sorts have poured out a stream of criticism, whose vehemence is often startling even to those who would themselves criticize the profession. Certainly criticism of doctors and their work is no new phenomenon. From the time of Plato's admonition to doctors not to prescribe medication or perform surgery without consulting adequately with their patients to that of Ambrose Bierce's definition of a doctor as someone "upon whom we set our hopes when ill and our dogs when well," there has been an ever-growing body of criticism directed at the medical establishment. What is new and noteworthy is that in midtwentieth-century America, the genre flourished at precisely the time that medical science reached its most advanced stage.[58]

Whereas medicine's more judicious critics attempt to write in an honest and level-headed response to serious problems, there are among their less judicious counterparts many who resort to emotionalism and misrepresentation. Yet the very vehemence that informs the writings of these less judicious critics points to an underlying sense of betrayal resulting, at least in part, from the violation of their own expectations. These writers, as does much of the public they address, appear to wreak vengeance upon those who seem to have betrayed them. The trend has not gone unnoticed. Shryock, writing as early as 1947, remarked that "for the recent decades, the real question was not whether the public acquired confidence in medicine, but whether they expected too much of it."[59] Echoing Shryock more than two decades later, economist Eli Ginzberg commented that "the question that is worth raising is what lies back of this recurrent crisis in American medicine? The answer seems to lie in the sudden wide gap that has been introduced between our expectations and our abilities to meet them."[60]

It is, then, expectations raised too high, expectations growing directly out of both the needed doctor-patient relationship and out of the myriad cultural representations of that relationship that are one of the root causes of the problems confronting American doctors and their patients. To begin to understand these expectations, their genesis, and evocative power, it is helpful to understand the process by which people come to expect certain things from the world around them. How people respond to the reality of their daily lives is a result of the interaction between the immediate experiences they have and the remembered past experiences, both actual and vicarious, that they carry with them. Out of this remembered and ever-present past are formed the expectations that help give shape and direction to the unfolding present. Thus, to know the ways in which the past lives on in the expectations of the present is to begin to know how a society, through its many creations, touches and influences the lives of all who are a part of it.

4

The Power of Expectations: Theoretical Frameworks

EXPECTATIONS AND SOCIALIZATION

Without expectations, people could not function. Without the ability to generalize from past experience in order to form expectations about future experience and to devise behaviors in response to that future, people would be forever re-establishing their worlds. If the nature of each recurring experience had to be verified, all of a person's time and energy would be consumed in testing the fabric of the most immediate and crucial of everyday experiences. Upon awakening, every morning of every day the individual would have to ask and answer countless questions: Will the bedroom floor be there? Will the bathroom faucet provide safe water? Will clothing fit as it did last night? Will eggs and toast taste the same as they did yesterday? Will the world outside the door remain familiar and provide the same stimuli it did before? Not until the answers to such questions were determined could the individual begin to go about the less basic of life's everyday activities.

For the majority of people, however, these and similar questions are never thought of, never asked. The answers have been learned as part of a person's generalized response to past experience. The floor will be there. The water will be safe. Clothing will fit. Breakfast will taste the same. The world outside the door will be familiar. Assuming without even thinking that their expectations about the basic components of their lives will be fulfilled, people venture beyond their front doors with confidence that their world will remain stable. Of course, that confidence can be shaken, but until it is called into question it provides a base of certainty, a learned response to life, upon which people can ground their activities.

This learning process is part of primary socialization, the first and most important form of the more general process of socialization that introduces the individual to the everyday, objective world of his or her society.[1] At the same time that socialization introduces the individual to the encompassing objective world and its demands, the process also, and more importantly, introduces the individual to the subjective world of selfhood. This phase of socialization is well-described by Peter L. Berger and Thomas Luckmann in *The Social Construction of Reality* as they demonstrate that

> the self is a reflected entity, reflecting the attitudes first taken [during primary socialization] by significant others toward it; the individual becomes what he is addressed as by his significant others. This is not a one-sided mechanistic process. It entails a dialectic between identification by others and self-identification, between objectively and subjectively appropriated identity.[2]

The process also entails a dialectic between the expectations of others and self-expectations. In short, the individual becomes in large part what others expect her or him to become.

During primary socialization, a child learns to abstract general rules and principles of behavior from the specific, ad hoc responses of significant others. What first one's parents, then siblings, then grandparents, and others respond to positively or negatively becomes, in time, part of the socialized individual's repertoire of responses to the world. In this way, the power of any norm (behaviors and expectations included) is generalized and subjectively extended.[3]

Once generalized, norms and the expectations upon which they are based can be accepted as integral parts of the individual's subjectively defined identity. The degree to which norms and expectations are accepted (or internalized) determines both the success of the socialization process *and* the success with which the individual becomes a functioning member of a particular social world. Once provided, via primary socialization, with a working script that spells out the patterns of behavior that are expected and acceptable, the individual is able to begin to cope with the fundamental experiences of life.

Having internalized expectations about and behavior patterns to follow in response to such basic activities as eating, toileting, and fearing or not fearing, the individual can move beyond primary socialization. During the maturational years when primary socialization gives way to secondary socialization, the individual is at risk for losing the psychic foundation provided by the never totally internalized dicta of primary socialization. Crucial here is "how the reality internalized in primary socialization is maintained in consciousness." Equally crucial to the individual's successful growth is "how further internalizations—or secondary socializations—take place."[4] An allied problem, whose solution is an integral part of everyone's life, is to maintain the portion of reality internalized during secondary socialization. Although intertwined, the two realities derived from the two different stages of socialization vary in their potency and tenacity. They also vary in the manner in which they are maintained in the individual's consciousness and behavior.

The psychic process of secondary socialization is similar to that of primary socialization, and expectations function in much the same way in both. Secondary socialization, however, introduces the individual to a less immediate and more escapable world, one that originates at a greater distance from the self than did the world first taken in during primary socialization. Depending as it does upon "the internalization of institutional or institution-based 'sub-worlds,' secondary socialization entails the acquisition of role specific knowledge."[5] In contrast, primary socialization can be seen as the acquisition of role general knowledge. All people come to know the ways of eating, sleeping, providing shelter, and reproducing. Only certain people come to know the ways of healing wounds, building cathedrals, or designing computer circuits. On the continuum ranging from the most exoteric to the most esoteric of life's experiences, the dividing line between primary and secondary socialization may shift at different times and in different places, but it is inevitably determined by the distinction between what all people and what only particular groups of people come to know and do.

Not only does secondary socialization introduce a person to less immediate and commonplace segments of reality, but it does so via agents that are less intimate with and less influential on a person.

> While primary socialization cannot take place without an emotionally charged identification with his [or her] significant others, most secondary socialization can dispense with this kind of identification and proceed effectively with only the amount of mutual identification that enters into any communication between human beings. Put crudely, it is necessary to love one's mother, but not one's teacher.[6]

From at least one theoretical perspective, it is possible to learn from but not love one's teacher precisely *because* at an earlier time one both loved and learned from one's mother (or equally significant other). The expectations about and behavior in response to learning situations that are engendered during primary socialization prepare the individual for the eventual move into more esoteric subworlds in which the agents of socialization are increasingly anonymous and institutionally defined. Having come to know him or herself via the expectations and behavior of significant others during childhood, the individual can come to define that self more fully and precisely via the expectations and responses of others who are increasingly less significant.

Because less influential agents operating within less immediate spheres of reality are the channels through which secondary socialization occurs, its effects are less deeply rooted and, hence, less inevitable than are the effects of primary socialization. The degree of inevitability also bears a direct relationship to the commonality of the particular segment of reality involved. The more central a given role and its attendant expectations and behavior patterns are to the individual's well-being, the less readily will the acquired knowledge about that role be called into question. It is not likely that a person will question whether the role of food-eater is necessary to well-being. It is possible, however, that having been socialized to a particular *mode* of eating behavior, a person may come to modify both the expectations about and the performance of that behavior when faced repeatedly with situations that demonstrate the ineffectiveness or inappropriateness of that particular form of internalized behavior.

CULTURE AND REALITY MAINTENANCE

It is possible that people might come to question their expectations about and behavior in response to the most fundamental of their daily activities. If food suddenly ceased to nourish, or if it inexplicably began to kill, or if a highly influential starvation cult rose to power, it is possible that eating would no longer be an unquestioned part of everyday life. Though extreme, the example does point to a continuous problem that all societies face. Because the operational dicta of primary and secondary socializations are never totally formed and never fully internalized, they are continually threatened in a changing world. In order to preserve these dicta, which are crucial to their survival, all societies have to "develop procedures of reality maintenance to safeguard a measure of symmetry between" people's internal and external worlds.[7] Without such symmetry, an individual would face the perpetual threat of irreparable tears in the fabric of everyday life, and the individual's encompassing world, the society of which she or he is a part, would face the perpetual threat of fragmentation and disintegration. In order to ward off such threats, individuals and the societies they comprise devise and share certain patterns of behavior that serve to maintain the reality of their everyday life.

The patterns of behavior that contribute to reality maintenance constitute a significant part of the culture of any particular society or interactional group. The pervasive and persuasive nature of culture is evident in Clyde Kluckhohn's brief definition of the abstraction: culture is "the total life way of a people, the social legacy the individual acquires from the group."[8] The shared, learned behaviors (in all their manifestations) from which a given culture can be inferred and described serve to perpetuate the group and its solidarity.[9] In other words, the way everybody does everything (to paraphrase Gertrude Stein) becomes, via its transmission, the means by which any society deals with the problem of reality maintenance.

To see *how* the shared learned behavior of a given society's culture functions to maintain the reality of what has been internalized during primary and secondary socialization, it is helpful to examine a more comprehensive definition of "culture," one set forth by Kluckhohn and Kroeber:

> Culture consists of patterns explicit and implicit, of and for behavior, acquired and transmitted by symbols constituting the distinctive achievement of human groups, including their embodiment in artifacts; the essential core of culture consists of traditional (i.e. historically derived and selected) ideas and especially their attached values; culture systems may, on the one hand, be considered as products of action, on the other as conditioning elements of further action.[10]

The most potent set of symbols by which behavior patterns are acquired and transmitted is language, the sine qua non of reality maintenance. The special power of language stems from its ability to objectify the world and to transform the constant flux of experience into a seemingly coherent and orderly pattern. While establishing that pattern, language functions in two crucial ways: it enables apprehension, *and* it provides the means by which people articulate what they apprehend.[11] Once able to name people, things, actions, ideas, and the like, an individual "knows of" and can begin to affirm and share the full range of life's experiences. Language, then, in its several forms makes possible and efficient the transmission of learned, shared, and expected behavior without which no culture could survive.

People experience language most immediately in conversation; thus, as Berger and Luckmann point out, conversation is "the most important vehicle of reality maintenance."[12] As such, conversation is also the most important vehicle for the transmission of a society's expectations about individual behavior in the broadest sense. Without the continuous stream of casual daily conversation, people would cease to know themselves, and they would begin to question the once taken-for-granted reality of their lives.

Any society, then, depends on the conversational form of language to maintain the ongoing reality of expectations and actions that give rise to the particular forms of behavior shared by its members. Without the language of conversation, there could be no culture, for without that form of language there would be no way to share and pass on the group's knowledge of and expectations about accepted modes of behavior.[13] All of the vital elements of a society—its remembered past, its expected future, its myriad ways of being and doing, in short, its culture—are brought into the life of each of its members by means of talk. Because people can talk, they can come to know and maintain their own self-identifications; they can come also to share and affirm the ongoing reality of the culture of their particular social world.

THE ROLE OF ARTIFACTS

The language of conversation makes possible the sharing and maintenance of culture in immediate, face-to-face situations. Similarly, the artifacts of a society enable people to share and maintain their culture regardless of temporal or spatial boundaries. The "made things" of a society allow people to converse in an extended dialogue that is hindered by neither time nor space. Artifacts arising from the experience of individuals at one place and time become a form of experience for other individuals at another place and time. As such they become, in the same way as do actual and immediate experience, a part of a society's remembered and articulated past, which lives on in and influences its ever-unfolding present of expectations and behavior.

Although artifacts of all types transmit and maintain the everyday reality of a people's culture, linguistic artifacts are especially important to the process because language is the most readily available and the most widely shared medium through which people can communicate about the realities of their lives. Dance, paintings, cooking utensils, sculpture, and other non-linguistic artifacts also spring from and in turn influence experience, but the apprehension and understanding of such cultural products always involves a linguistic transformation of a given artifact into an analogous form of verbal explanation—that dance expresses joy; that wall painting conveys the exhilaration of the hunt; that bowl shows pride. Nonlinguistic artifacts become fully a part of people's lives through the shared understandings made possible by language; linguistic artifacts, because they are more immediately available to people, are more readily able to transmit and maintain a culture.

The centrality of linguistic artifacts is also a result of what Berger and Luckmann call the "detachability" of language. Although first generated in personal encounters, language can exist without and beyond them. Via memory, writing, and electronic media, words can be detached from the immediately personal sphere. Further,

> the detachment of language lies more basically in its capacity to communicate meanings that are not direct expressions of subjectivity "here and now." It shares this capacity with other sign systems, but its immense variety and complexity make it much more readily detachable from the face-to-face situation than any other...I can speak about innumerable matters that...I never have and never will experience directly. In this way, language is capable of becoming the objective repository of vast accumulations of meaning and experience, which it can preserve in time and transmit to following generations.[14]

The "accumulations of meaning and experience" that language contains are preserved and transmitted more completely and efficiently in linguistic artifacts than in immediate conversation. Such artifacts, therefore, are crucial to the survival of any culture. The daily talk of men and women passes quickly from a society's grasp, but its linguistic artifacts, tangible and preserved, form an indestructible bridge across which the expectations and desired behavior of a society can move. Without such artifacts, a society's task of reality maintenance would be far more difficult and the survival of its culture would be far less readily assured.

Because artifacts (both linguistic and nonlinguistic) enable people "to learn, to communicate by a system of learned symbols, and to transmit learned behavior from generation to generation," they are a product of what Kluckhohn describes as the very "characteristics of the human animal which make culture possible."[15] Given their crucial role in the genesis and maintenance of culture, the artifacts of any society can provide a means of seeing how people perceive and articulate the reality of their everyday lives. How people construct their worlds and how they transmit these constructions and reconstructions of reality both determine and are determined by the nature of their culture. This continuous interplay is similar to and in part a result of the interplay between people's expectations and their behavior, both of which can be examined via the manifest form they take in artifacts and action.

Although behavior is more easily described than are expectations, it would be wrong to conclude that the study of behavior is a more precise gauge of a people's culture than is a study of their expectations. Sociologist Richard Sykes addresses this question when he notes that "in culture studies *we are not exploring the real world, but rather what people believe about the real world*. We do not study behavior, but beliefs about behavior."[16] To study expectations, then is to come to know one of the determining factors that influence beliefs about behavior and behavior itself. Artifacts, because they arise from and in turn influence expectations, can provide insight into the expectations that people hold about the workings of their world and about the ways in which men and women do and ought to perform in that world.

TO WHAT EFFECT

To assert that artifacts play a crucial role in the dialectic between people's expectations and their behavior is to assume that cultural products do have a demonstrable effect on the mental lives of those who experience them. That assumption, crucial as it is, deserves further examination. The question of the effect of any cultural form and its *transmission* was given its classic formulation in 1947 in H. D. Laswell's description of the communication process as "Who says what to whom, how, and with what effect."[17] Since then, effect studies have been a particular concern of communications researchers whose findings can illuminate the interrelationships among artifacts, language, expectations, and behavior.

An early proposition, elaborating on Laswell and useful in setting the parameters within which the overall question of effects would have to be addressed, was Bernard Berelson's statement that "Some kinds of communication, brought to the attention of some kinds of people under some kinds of conditions, have some kinds of effects."[18] Prototypic in its root assertion that the mass media (and by extension all cultural artifacts) do affect people, Berelson's proposition was also prototypic in suggesting the difficulties involved in pinpointing those effects and assigning them with any degree of certainty to particular causes. Over the years, communications researchers have faced these difficulties with varying degrees of success.[19] Characteristically, after compiling a list of thirty-two hypotheses that reflected the state of communications research in the late 1940s, Wilbur Schramm was able to conclude only that research could yield little because of the difficulties involved in isolating cause and effect in a complex environmental process.[20]

The frustrations of researchers were aggravated by public disenchantment, pointed to in Joseph T. Klapper's description of the field in 1960: "It is surely no wonder that a bewildered public should regard with cynicism a research tradition which supplies, instead of definitive answers, a plethora of relevant but inconclusive and at times seemingly contradictory findings." Klapper's own work, in which he proposed a phenomenistic approach that would attempt to take into account all interacting variables, only compounded the problem. Realizing this difficulty, he attempted to justify his own call for ever-more complex research by maintaining that although answers might be slower in coming, they would, in the end, be "more meaningful."[21]

One of the answers to which Klapper's work pointed was that mass communications ordinarily function among a complex of other factors and influences and are, therefore, contributory rather than causal agents. By setting the media into their broader cultural context, Klapper was able to reassert the complexity of the processes involved in the formation of expectations, attitudes, and behavior. No longer could effect studies proceed to view the sender, the receiver, and the message in isolation. Theoretical views of the communication process grew in breadth and sophistication so that researchers came to deal with sender, receiver, and message as well as with the sender's motives, the receiver's responses, the background of both of them, the origins and nature of interference, and its influence on the effectiveness of the message being transmitted.[22]

The debate about whether the mass media, and in fact all other cultural artifacts, are causal or only contributory factors has gone unresolved, largely because the distinction it poses is less important than other issues facing communications researchers. One such issue is the fact that apparently the mass media tend to reinforce preexisting attitudes rather than change them significantly.[23] This tendency for the media to act as agents of reinforcement rather than change is explained well by Walter Weiss, who has determined that people will watch (or listen to or read) what they want to for certain rewards:

> Since there is need to attract and hold an audience, the media cannot vary too much from the audience's expectations or values or desires. Hence, the media tend to reflect current characteristics of people and, by reinforcing them, act as a conservative influence ... In other words, a significant portion of the total outcome of communications experience is the reinforcement or intensification or elicitation of preexisting responses.[24]

As persuasive as they are about the conservative influence exerted by the mass media in particular and by all artifacts in general, neither Klapper nor Weiss is willing to address the question of where the "current characteristics" and "preexisting responses" originate. That question has no ready answer. Any audience's "expectations or values or desires," as well as their beliefs and modes of being, are made up of an endlessly receding chain of experiences handed down from parent to child, generation after generation, via the sharing made possible by cultural transmission. There is no way to determine first causes. As a result, all factors in the remembered past, the lived present, and the anticipated future must be considered as contributing to the mental lives of the members of any given society.

Because language is such a potent force, linguistic artifacts hold a special place among the many made things that influence people's lives, a place that compels close examination of a culture's linguistic creations. Also (and here it is important to keep in mind Sykes' assertion that culture studies are concerned with both actual *and* perceived reality), linguistic artifacts can provide access to both of these forms of reality. The language of history and sociology can present an approximation of reality as it may have been, whereas the language of novels, movies, television shows, and such can demonstrate much about the perceived reality of the makers of artifacts and their audience.

Also, since there is a constant interplay between the actual and the perceived, the artifacts of any society are more than just the products of certain people's responses to their worlds. Artifacts that arise out of historical forces and circumstances contribute to people's views of those circumstances and of themselves and their past and present worlds. Touched by that web of experience—past and present, actual and transformed—people come to expect certain things about themselves and their worlds. What they expect influences what they are and what they do, which in turn influences the shape and texture of the culture they make and share.

DOCTORS AND PATIENTS

The real power of expectations, then, stems from their ability to influence as well as reflect mental states and behavior patterns. Thus to know the nature of people's expectations is to begin to understand the dynamic interplay between historical reality and people's responses to it. Those responses, when embodied in cultural artifacts, are available for examination long after a particular artificer or a particular set of circumstances has passed from the immediate scene. Artifacts live to tell their tale long after the forces that gave rise to them are gone from view. With careful handling, artifacts from the past can reveal much about the interrelationships among experience, expectations, and behavior as well as the effects of all of those factors on a people's culture.

To understand all of this is to see how a generalized attitude toward and certain expectations about doctors in America could grow out of human wants, historical circumstances, and the artifacts that sprang from and reflected those. Not until the last third of the nineteenth century could patients reasonably expect very much from their doctors. Patients could expect, and more often than not did receive, moral support and comfort during times of personal and family crisis. Far less often did they receive truly efficacious care; the state of medical knowledge and practice simply did not allow that. Although there is no way to date precisely the time at which attitudes and expectations began to grow more positive, such a change could not have occurred until the reality of improved medical practice allowed the minimal level of competence necessary to promote, among patients, a modicum of trust and hope. Laying the foundations for that minimal level of competence were the actual accomplishments of medical science and the perceptions of those accomplishments by people who, on a wide scale, came to expect similar improvements in the day-to-day medical care they received.

Once the medical profession was able to do more, people could expect more in spite of any lingering doubts they might have held. Once people's expectations grew more positive, those expectations were reflected in the artifacts that became one way of sharing and handing down beliefs and hopes about the nature and effectiveness of health care. Because the maintenance of health and life is such a basic concern, what is learned about doctors and about the doctor-patient relationship exerts considerable influence on all concerned. Thus the expectations that arise out of actual and vicarious experience are very fully internalized, even though these expectations occur during the period of secondary socialization when what is internalized is always open to later modification.

As American medicine was able to provide more and better care through the first decades of the twentieth century,[25] expectations about that care not only kept pace with but eventually outdistanced the reality of what the profession could do. As America's idealized image of the doctor grew and took hold, the health care system was actually beginning to suffer from the inability to continue doing what people more and more expected it to do. In the disparity between image and reality lay the seeds of discontent that remained dormant until midcentury. Not until then were the expectations of enough people violated often enough for the internalized image of doctors and their work to be called seriously into question.[26]

Ironically, and in spite of ever-increasing attacks on the health care system, the image of the doctor in America continues in large part to be an idealization that reflects people's hopes rather than their actual experiences. To see the origins of that idealization and to understand the hold it exerts on people, the next four chapters examine a sampling of the artifacts that have contributed to the socially constructed version of an ideal that is not only out of touch with everyday reality but is actually a detriment to and a problem for doctors and patients alike.

5

Literary Artifacts: Origins

THE PERVASIVE IMAGE: FROM "LITERATURE" TO PULP

America's novelists have created a vast gallery of fictional doctors, most of them highly idealized characters, imbued with the twin virtues of rugged individualism and godlike omnipotence. In terms of numbers alone, novels about doctors or novels in which doctors play a prominent role, are noteworthy. Evelyn Rivers Wilbanks, in her admittedly incomplete checklist, "The Physician in the American Novel, 1870–1955," lists 381 novels that "focus on a physician as the main character." The list, arbitrarily restricted "to confine the material to a workable scope,"[1] excludes the novels of Charles Brockden Brown, Nathaniel Hawthorne, and Oliver Wendell Holmes, all of whom created physicians of widely different types prior to Wilbanks's starting date of 1870. The checklist, which ends in 1955, does not include the continuous stream of "doctor novels" that has appeared since the 1950s. A complete list (if such were possible) would likely double Wilbanks's tally.

Not only are the portrayals of doctors numerically significant, but, more importantly, they also range in quality from memorable art to mere pulp. Doctors appear as significant characters in the novels and shorter fiction of America's "best" writers—among them Nathaniel Hawthorne, Henry James, Sherwood Anderson, Sinclair Lewis, William Faulkner, and F. Scott Fitzgerald—as well as in the outpourings of the masters of pulp whose fiction is rapidly digested by its mass audience. Between these extremes of "best" and "worst" lies another large body of fiction by America's lesser-rank novelists—William Dean Howells, Sarah Orne Jewett, John O'Hara, Carson McCullers, and the like—as well as by that varied lot of writers whose novels have come to be known either statistically or by reputation as "best-sellers." The idealized image is evident in all of these types. Thus it has been and remains available to all segments of the American reading public. Because "the doctor" has been so frequently a subject of the novelist's work and because the portrayals that embody the evolving image of the American doctor have been so widely distributed throughout the reading public, the novel is a particularly useful artifact to examine in an attempt to assess the cultural forces that have helped form the image of the doctor presented to the American public.

The novel's usefulness in this regard is heightened by its other characteristics as well. Unlike shorter fiction, the novel works on a broader canvas, which allows a more detailed and extensive presentation of character and milieu. Unlike drama, which, in both its written and staged forms, reaches a limited audience, the novel has a far broader public, hence (at least potentially) a far greater inherent power to mold expectations and influence behavior. Furthermore, unlike nonfiction prose, the novel is more likely to embody both a sense of historical place and attitude as well as a delineation of behavior both expressed and expected.

Previous studies of the doctor's portrayal in American literature do take note of the establishment of an idealized image, but the task remains to elaborate on the cultural implications of the artifacts they examine. Lois Elizabeth DeBakey's unpublished dissertation, "The Physician-scientist as Character in Nineteenth Century American Literature," surveys the fiction of Hawthorne, Herman Melville, Oliver Wendell Holmes, S. Weir Mitchell, Howells, and Jewett, and asserts that the literature of the period "presents a fairly accurate picture of the profession during that era."[2] DeBakey concludes that "the most skillful creative artists disparage the physician while less gifted writers flatter him."[3]

Reaching similar conclusions is William M. Marchand's "The Changing Role of the Medical Doctor in Selected Plays in American Drama." Marchand, like DeBakey, does not account for the complex interrelationships among writer, audience, and the encompassing cultural milieu. Rather, he summarizes the historical evolution of the stage-doctor and reaches his final claim: "It is to the credit of the medical profession that the bulk of American fiction [sic] using the doctor as a character finds reason to praise him."[4] More recent and briefer attempts to deal with the doctor as a literary type examine a smattering of portrayals and note that doctors are painted as both romantic heroes and scapegoats[5]; though their studies are useful, the writers do not attempt to reconcile these polar opposites or to set them into a broader historical and cultural framework.

This broader cultural and chronological framework must be kept in mind if these artifacts are to be viewed accurately and understood fully. Also, given the pervasiveness of the idealized doctor in America's literary canon, it is useful to survey the several types of fictional portrayals. The discussion that follows deals with the "best" and the "worst" of American fiction as well as with that broad middle ground filled with best-sellers and the works of minor novelists. Because such an inquiry is potentially endless in scope and in order to alleviate the excesses resulting from a comprehensive survey, representative and accessible works from each of several types are examined and stand for the rest of their kind. Also, the literary artifacts examined do not range through the whole of American literature; rather, they start with the fiction of Hawthorne since prior to that, American novelists produced few memorable doctors.[6] Beginning with Hawthorne, however, writers came more and more to include the doctor as an integral member of their fictional worlds.

Starting off with Hawthorne offers the additional advantage of establishing a beginning point that coincides with the time period in which the American medical profession began to police its own ranks and to set into motion the improvements that would so dramatically change it in the last decade of the nineteenth century. Hawthorne published *The Scarlet Letter* in 1850, four years after the appearance of *Mosses From An Old Manse*, which presented two of his most memorable doctors, Aylmer and Rappaccini. Between those years, the American Medical Association was founded, and the image established by Hawthorne's physicians changed rapidly in the novels of the next decades in ways similar to the changes occurring within the medical profession itself. To begin with Hawthorne's physicians is to step into fictional worlds far different from those created by his followers. To do so is also to pose a striking counterpoint against which the image that would evolve in the ensuing decades can be seen in even clearer outlines as an idealization, at first keeping pace with and then far outstripping the reality of the medical and social worlds from which it sprang.

HAWTHORNE'S DOCTORS: THE NADIR OF THE IMAGE

Hawthorne's doctors and scientists practice the art of healing within fictional worlds that both admire and fear what they do. This ambivalence is similar to what was felt by Americans toward their own doctors during the decades when Hawthorne wrote. Ironically, the capabilities of Hawthorne's fictional doctors far exceeded what doctors actually could do in the midnineteenth century. Yet in their very abilities lie the seeds of the downfall of these fictional healers, a downfall used repeatedly by Hawthorne to explore the broader issues of the limits of human knowledge and the consequences attendant upon reaching beyond those limits. In their overreaching, Hawthorne's doctors inevitably sunder themselves from humanity and enact a ritualized pattern that points to the root cause of the distrust (both fictional and real) of the doctor's expertise. In his fiction, Hawthorne speaks pointedly of the ambivalence toward expertise that is an inevitable part of the doctor-patient relationship. While giving little overt attention to explaining the origins of this ambivalence, Hawthorne manages to provide insight into its very roots by showing the machinations of doctors who invariably pervert their potential for good into a stark actualization of evil.

Although the evil wrought by Hawthorne's doctors takes different forms, it is always a variation of the Unpardonable Sin sought for and described explicitly by the title character of the tale "Ethan Brand." Doctor to the mind and intellectual wanderer, Brand had set forth on a quest for "the image of some mode of guilt which could neither be atoned for nor forgiven."[7] After years of worldwide searching, he returns to the lime-kiln where he had begun his quest. Once there, he describes the Unpardonable Sin, saying, " 'It is a sin that grew within my own breast . . . A sin that grew nowhere else! The sin of an intellect that triumphed over the sense of brotherhood with man and reverence for God, and sacrificed everything to its own mighty claims. The only sin that deserves a recompense of immortal agony!' " (p. 306).

Brand's answer embodies Hawthorne's concern with the problem of the intellect that oversteps its natural boundaries and in so doing precipitates disaster. Later in the tale, the narrative gives a more complete and dispassionate explication of Brand's sin, which had its origins in genuine "love and sympathy for mankind and . . . pity for human guilt and woe." From this concern grew the inspiration that became Brand's obsession, and from his search for the Unpardonable Sin "ensued that vast intellectual development, which, in its progress disturbed the counterpoise between his mind and heart" (pp. 313–14). Once that counterpoise was disturbed, there followed a growth of intellect that made Brand the envy of the philosophers of the earth while it paved the way for his downfall.

The tale's narrator grants Brand's intellectual eminence, but he also questions it in a passage crucial to an understanding of Hawthorne's moral vision and his recurrent use of the doctor-scientist as the prototype of the person who disturbs the proper balance between mind and heart:

> So much for the intellect! But where was the heart? That, indeed, had withered,—had contracted,—had hardened,—had perished! It had ceased to partake of the universal throb. He had lost his hold on the magnetic chain of humanity. He was no longer a brother-man, opening the chambers or the dungeons of our common nature by the key of holy sympathy, which gave him a right to share in all its secrets; he was now a cold observer, looking on mankind as the subject of his experiment, and, at length converting man and woman to be his puppets, and pulling the wires that moved them to such degrees of crime as were demanded for his study.
>
> Thus Ethan Brand became a fiend. He began to be so from the moment

that his moral nature had ceased to keep pace of improvement with his intellect. (p. 314)

This explicit account of Brand's transformation anticipates Hawthorne's archetypal fiend, Chillingworth, just as it further illuminates the fiendish nature of both Aylmer and Rappaccini, the earlier embodiments of doctors whose powers were turned ultimately to destructive ends. These three doctors exemplify more subtly and in more artistically successful ways the essential image of the overreacher-as-destroyer that is presented explicitly and didactically in "Ethan Brand." Hawthorne's short fiction is both well known enough and of such quality that its inclusion here is important, even though the focus is on novelistic treatments of the doctor. Furthermore, the tales of Aylmer and Rappaccini as well as that of Ethan Brand provide a way of viewing the development of Chillingworth as a character who grew from earlier, less completely realized portrayals.

In "The Birthmark," Hawthorne portrays a doctor who aspires to the ultimate goal of his profession, attaining perfection by eradicating illness and death. The metaphoric construct that Hawthorne uses is the attempt by Aylmer, the consummate man of science, to remove a small hand-shaped birthmark from the cheek of his otherwise ideally beautiful wife, Georgianna. Though trivial to the objective eye, the birthmark becomes, for Aylmer and for Georgianna (and eventually for the reader), a potent symbol of humanity's susceptibility to disease and inevitable death, the ultimate forms of earthly imperfection. That such imperfection is inherent in the human state is ignored by Aylmer, whose expertise and pride blind him to the dangers involved in tampering with nature's ordained cycle. His overreaching pride and intellect are evident as he reassures Georgianna of his ability to remove the birthmark and as he comments confidently, " 'What will be my trimuph when I shall have corrected what Nature left imperfect in her fairest work! Even Pygmalion, when his sculptured woman assumed life felt not greater ecstasy than mine will be.' "[8]

Neither ecstasy nor success, though, is to be Aylmer's lot. Unable to accept human fallibility and limitation, he blinds himself to the fact that what he will attempt is a transgression of the natural order of things. He deludes himself and his wife as he says, reassuringly, " 'I would not wrong either you or myself by working such inharmonious effects upon our lives; but I would have you consider how trifling, in comparison, is the skill requisite to remove this little hand' " (p. 212). That skill, though, is far greater than he had anticipated and, finally, more than he can muster in his quest for perfection. What happens to Aylmer as he works his experiment on Georgianna is what has already happened to him repeatedly in his earlier and most lofty endeavors: his own ineludible humanity subverts and finally destroys his highest aspirations.

Aylmer's attempt to transcend the clay—the mortality and earthly imperfection—of the human state leads to his ultimate failure and to the destruction of Georgianna. In his overreaching, Aylmer, as did Ethan Brand, loses hold of the magnetic chain of humanity; so, too, does he tear Georgianna from her own rightful place in that chain. In consequence, he attains a momentary success that turns quickly into total failure. As the hated birthmark fades from her cheek, Georgianna dies: "Thus ever does the gross fatality of earth exult in its invariable triumph over the immortal essence which, in this dim sphere of half development, demands the completeness of a higher state." By trying to reach that unattainable "higher state," Aylmer rejects, as Georgianna tells him in her dying words, " 'the best the earth could offer' " (p. 220). Her death, the result of Aylmer's misuse of his powers, is a potent warning about the dangers inherent in reaching beyond one's human state.

Hawthorne's concern with the overreacher who rejects what is fundamentally human and in consequence breaks the magnetic chain of humanity is most fully rendered in "Rappaccini's Daughter." Here the overreacher is Signor Giacomo Rappaccini, "the famous doctor, who . . . it is said . . . distills plants into medicines that are as potent as a charm."[9] The tale of Rappaccini is richer and more consciously romantic than that of Aylmer, mainly because Hawthorne manipulates the point of view to establish an air of ambiguity in regard to Rappaccini's activities, thereby allowing the tale to comment on the nature of perception and shared guilt as well as on the consequences of using knowledge and expertise to malevolent ends. Rappaccini has spent his life and dedicated his skill to the cultivation and perfection of vegetable poisons possessed, or so he believes, of medicinal properties. In his pursuits he has enlisted the aid of his daughter Beatrice, whom he has kept in virtual seclusion in the garden that she helps him tend. Intruding upon this Edenic scene comes Giovanni Guasconti, newly arrived to study at the University of Padua, who takes lodging in rooms overlooking the garden. Giovanni's introduction into the garden sets in motion the events that bring about the downfall of Rappaccini and the death of the innocent Beatrice.

Hawthorne's third-person narrative is filtered largely through the perceptions of Giovanni, and the narrator takes great pains to call into question the accuracy and validity of what the impressionable young man *thinks* he sees in his encounters with Beatrice, with Rappaccini, and with the luxuriant garden. The increasingly ambiguous nature of Giovanni's vision echoes the moral ambiguity that is one of the tale's central concerns. Furthermore, the uncertain nature of Giovanni's perceptions and judgments forces the reader finally to decide about the nature and true source of the evil that destroys Beatrice. From the very first, Giovanni is characterized as an unreliable observer whose lively imagination and natural "tendency to heartbreak" lead him to interpret what he sees in terms fraught with evil implications. Looking down upon Rappaccini tending his garden, the young man is impressed "most disagreeably; for the man's demeanor was that of one walking among malignant influences... which, should he allow them one moment of license, would wreak upon him some terrible fatality." In contrast to Giovanni's fearful view is that of the more neutral narrative voice that moves back from what the young man has seen and comments, "It was strangely frightful to the young man's *imagination* [emphasis added] to see the air of insecurity in a person cultivating a garden, that most simple and innocent of human toils" (p. 270).

Hawthorne's narrative strategy here is to keep the tale located continually in that "neutral territory, somewhere between the real world and fairy-land, where the Actual and the Imaginary may meet and each imbue itself with the nature of the other."[10] By doing this, he is able to postpone the reader's final judgment and to provide dual explanations for the events presented. Just as Giovanni's views of Rappaccini and the garden are qualified, so, too, is his initial reaction to Beatrice presented in a manner that forces the reader to defer judgment about her. When she appears, in the day's waning light, the narrative voice describes her as Giovanni sees her: "Soon there emerged from under a sculptured portal the figure of a young girl, arrayed with as much richness of taste as the most splendid of the flowers, beautiful as the day, and with a bloom so deep and vivid that one shade more would have been too much. She looked redundant with life, health, and energy" (p. 271). Seeing what Giovanni sees, the reader is immediately given both the young man's subjective response to Beatrice and the narrator's view of that response: "Yet Giovanni's fancy must have grown morbid while he looked down into the garden; for the impression which the fair stranger made upon him was as if here were another flower, the human sister of those vegetable ones, as beautiful as they, more beautiful than the richest of them, but still to be touched only with a glove, nor to be approached without a mask" (p. 271).

The likely morbidity of Giovanni's fancy is re-emphasized in the description of his reactions on the morning following his first view of Beatrice and her father. With characteristic ambiguity, Hawthorne introduces a more commonplace view made possible by "the light of morning that tends to rectify whatever errors of fancy, or even of judgment, we may have incurred during the sun's decline, or among the shadows of the night, or in the less wholesome glow of moonlight" (p. 272). In the light of day, Giovanni sees things differently: "the garden which his dreams had made so fertile of mysteries...[is now a] real and matter-of-fact...affair...in the first rays of the sun...[it is] brought within the limits of ordinary experience." In the light of a new day, Giovanni is "inclined to take a most rational view of the whole matter" (p. 272). Yet, for the reader who has been led to suspect the young man's perceptions, Giovanni's "rational view" is, ironically, no more reliable than the fanciful one it has replaced.

A seemingly more complete view of Rappaccini is soon presented to Giovanni by Signoir Pietro Baglioni, "professor of medicine in the university, a physician of eminent repute to whom Giovanni had brought a letter of introduction" (p. 273). Giovanni asks Baglioni about the keeper of the strange garden, and to his surprise, Baglioni responds with a warning and a somber explanation of Rappaccini's work. Baglioni grants that Rappaccini is "eminently skilled" and has as much science as any number of the faculty—with perhaps one single exception—in Padua or all Italy," but then he goes on to qualify this praise by noting that "there are certain grave objections to his professional character" (p. 273). Pressed by Giovanni for more details, Baglioni explains Rappaccini in a way that seems to place him among Hawthorne's other unpardonable sinners, men whose obsessive quests have taken them from their place in the human community: " ' . . . he cares infinitely more for science than for mankind. His patients are interesting to him only as subjects for some new experiment. He would sacrifice human life, his own among the rest, or whatever was dearest to him, for the sake of adding so much as a grain of mustard to the great heap of his accumulated knowledge' " (p. 274).

Having presented his negative view, Baglioni continues with his characterization of Rappaccini in a way that begins to cast doubt on the objectivity and reliability of what he has already detailed. Baglioni insists that Rappaccini be held fully responsible for his failures, yet not be accorded full praise for his successes. The enmity hinted at here is made explicit as the narrative voice interjects and presents objective evidence of Baglioni's biased view: "The youth might have taken Baglioni's opinions with many grains of allowance had he known that there was a professional warfare of long continuance between him and Dr. Rappaccini, in which the latter was generally thought to have gained the advantage" (p. 274).

The grains of allowance, then, with which Giovanni should accept Baglioni's opinions are the same grains of allowance with which the reader comes to accept all that is presented in the tale in order, finally, to come to an accurate judgment about the varying degrees of guilt shared by the three men responsible for Beatrice's death. The nature and degree of their guilt place Giovanni, Baglioni, and Rappaccini squarely among Hawthorne's other unpardonable sinners and give to their activities an unprecedented cruelty, as each in turn victimizes the innocent Beatrice.

The cruelest victimizer is Rappaccini. The initially ambiguous view of his activities, presented through the skewed perceptions of Giovanni and the biased testimony of Baglioni, is systematically replaced by a clearer and finally more damning vision of him as the tale unfolds. In pursuit of his own ends, Rappaccini isolates his daughter from the rest of humanity and, worse, imbues her with the deadliest of poisons in order to verify his theories. Although not responsible for Giovanni's entrance into the garden, Rappaccini readily exploits the love that grows between the young man and Beatrice. Just as Ethan Brand and Aylmer had done, Rappaccini becomes a fiend whose moral nature ceases to keep pace with his intellectual achievements;

he is the "cold observer" who values others only as they can advance his own quest for knowledge. That he is responsible for making puppets of both Beatrice and Giovanni is clear in the tale's closing scene when Rappaccini enters the garden to watch the young lovers:

> As he drew near, the pale man of science seemed to gaze with a triumphal expression at the beautiful youth and maiden, as might an artist who should spend his life in achieving a picture or a group of statuary and finally be satisfied with his success. He paused; his bent form grew erect with conscious power; he spread out his hands over them in the attitude of a father imploring a blessing upon his children; but those were the same hands that had thrown poison into the stream of their lives. (p. 298)

At this point, Hawthorne ceases to present Rappaccini in a qualified manner; in direct and dramatic terms, Rappaccini's own words describe explicitly the evil he has wrought by removing Beatrice and Giovanni from the human community.

> "My daughter," said Rappaccini, "thou art no longer lonely in the world. Pluck one of those precious gems from thy sister shrub and bid thy bridegroom wear it in his bosom. It will not harm him now. My science and the sympathy between thee and him have so wrought within his system that he now stands apart from common men, as thou dost, daughter of my pride and triumph, from ordinary women. Pass on, then, through the world, most dear to one another and dreadful to all besides!" (p. 298)

Questioned by Beatrice about why he has subjected her to such a "miserable doom," Rappaccini presents the rationale for his actions. " 'Miserable!' exclaimed Rappaccini. 'What mean you, foolish girl? Dost thou deem it misery to be endowed with marvelous gifts against which no power nor strength could avail an enemy—misery, to be able to quell the mightiest with a breath—misery, to be as terrible as thou art beautiful? Wouldst thou, then, have preferred the condition of weak women, exposed to all evil and capable of none?' " In response to these impassioned questions, Beatrice says, simply, " 'I would have fain been loved, not feared' " (p. 298). In her dying cry for the most fundamental of human emotions, Beatrice destroys the illusion of Rappaccini's triumph and fully indicts her father for what he has done.

Rappaccini's deadly experiment epitomizes the vast disparity between his potential for good and his actualization of evil. Because of this he becomes the Unpardonable Sinner who has dedicated his skill and wisdom to perverted ends and has lost sight of his responsibility to and his place among humankind. Having negated his potential for good, Rappaccini objectifies the ever-present threat that the man of expertise may run amuck and flagrantly disregard the responsibility placed upon him by virtue of the very skill and power he comes to abuse.

This abuse of power and the perversion of the doctor's expertise are explored most fully by Hawthorne in *The Scarlet Letter*. Here, in the character of Roger Chillingworth, Hawthorne presents his most complex portrait of a healer who becomes the unpardonable sinner by dedicating his knowledge and skill to the achievement of malevolent ends, namely personal revenge. In the pursuit of that revenge, Chillingworth transforms himself from a needed agent of good into an embittered fiend who manipulates the lives of others and violates their essential humanity.

In the characterization of Chillingworth, Hawthorne takes care to establish the self-taught doctor's skill and potential for good. Intent upon discovering the identity of the man who has cuckolded him and fathered Hester Prynne's illegitimate child, Chillingworth swears his dishonored wife to silence about their relationship so that he may assume a new identity and enact his vendetta. The description of this new identity shows that the doctor is both needed and readily accepted as a potential boon to the community: " . . . it was as a physician that he presented himself, and as such was cordially received. Skilful [sic] men, of the medical and chirurgical profession, were of rare occurrence in the colony. . . . To such a professional body Roger Chillingworth was a brilliant acquisition."[11]

Having established this new identity, Chillingworth, "exemplary, as regarded at least the outward forms of a religious life" (p. 114), chooses the Reverend Arthur Dimmesdale as his spiritual advisor, unaware initially that Dimmesdale is the very man he has vowed to discover. Chillingworth's interest is first stirred by the minister's failing health, the physical manifestation of the spiritual malaise caused by his inability to confess his adulterous affair with Hester Prynne. Agonizing over his own guilt, Dimmesdale refuses the doctor's care at first, but finally he is persuaded to care for himself, and he agrees to confer with the physician. Thus, ironically, at the urging and with the approval of the community, the avenger becomes the physician and confidant of the man who is the subject of his search.

Between Chillingworth and Dimmesdale there soon grows the kind of intimate rapport both essential for effective treatment and one of the causes of the inevitable distrust that undergirds such a relationship. In simplest terms, the more the physician comes to know, the more potential power he has over the patient. As Hawthorne presents the relationship in its initial stages, he takes care to indicate that Chillingworth is still a benevolent healer; at the same time, the description makes amply clear that the very intimacy of the relationship will provide the means for Chillingworth to exact his revenge and, in the process, become the paradigm of the unpardonable sinner. In the manner of any careful diagnostician, Chillingworth "deemed it essential, it would seem, to know the man, before attempting to do him good" (p. 118).

In the course of his diagnostic probing, Chillingworth discovers Dimmesdale's secret, and in vowing to have revenge on his patient, the doctor, once benevolent, becomes a fiend in much the same way as had Ethan Brand. Having changed from the worthy healer to the cold observer, the aptly named Chillingworth decides on a form of revenge that can be achieved only by virtue of his role as healer-confidant:

> this unfortunate old man ... [came] to imagine a more intimate revenge than any mortal had ever wreaked upon an enemy. To make himself the one trusted friend, to whom should be confided all the fear, the remorse, the agony, the ineffectual repentence, the backward rush of sinful thoughts, expelled in vain! All that guilty sorrow, hidden from the world, whose great heart would have pitied and forgiven, to be revealed to him, the Pitiless, to him the Unforgiving! All that dark treasure to be lavished on the very man, to whom nothing else could so adequately pay the debt of vengeance. (pp. 133–134)

As perverse as Chillingworth's revenge appears to be, it is a revenge about which no easy judgment is allowed, for Hawthorne is concerned with the destructive effects of such malevolence on both its initiator and on its object. Soon after describing the form that Chillingworth's revenge will take, Hawthorne's narrator carefully presents what can be construed only as a sympathetic comment about the avenger, calling him a "poor, forlorn creature ... more wretched than his victim" (p. 135). The element of sympathy introduced here functions in much the same way as did the ambiguous portrayal of Rappaccini, forcing the reader to defer final judgment of Chillingworth until all of the evidence is presented.

Even more compelling than the partially sympathetic view hinted at by the narrative voice is the exchange between Hester and the physician in which Chillingworth reveals his own awareness of what his vengeance has cost him. Acknowledging his devilish manipulation of Dimmesdale, the old man gloats as he tells Hester that he must keep the minister alive in order to torture him:

> "Better had he died at once! Never did mortal suffer what this man has suffered. And all, all in the sight of his worst enemy! He had been conscious of me. He has felt an influence dwelling always upon him like a curse. He knew, by some spiritual sense,—for the Creator never made another being so sensitive as this,—he knew that no friendly hand was pulling at his heartstrings, and that an eye was looking curiously into him, which sought only evil, and found it." (p. 163)

Further admitting that his own life has come to be sustained "only by this perpetual poison of the direst revenge," Chillingworth concludes his self-indictment with words of anguished self-awareness: " 'Yea, indeed!—

he did not err!—there was a fiend at his elbow! A mortal man, with once a human heart, has become a fiend for his especial torment!' " (p. 163).

It is the tormentor's self-awareness that allows Hawthorne to refer, without ironic intent, to Chillingworth as "the unfortunate physician" at the very moment he recognizes the enormity of his own sin. Fully aware of what he has become, Chillingworth describes to Hester the transformation that has been wrought in him by the quest for revenge:

> "Dost thou remember me, Hester, as I was nine years agone? Even then, I was in the autumn of my days, nor was it an early autumn. But all my life had been made up of earnest, studious, thoughtful, quiet years, bestowed faithfully for the increase of mine own knowledge, and faithfully, too, though this latter object was but casual to the other,—faithfully for the advancement of human welfare. No life had been more peaceful and innocent than mine; few lives so rich with benefits conferred. Dost thou remember me? Was I not, though you might deem me cold, nevertheless a man thoughtful for others, craving little for himself,—kind, true, just, and of constant, if not warm affections? Was I not all this?"
>
> "All this, and more," said Hester.
>
> "And what am I now?" demanded he, looking into her face, and permitting the whole evil within him to be written on his features. "I have already told thee what I am! A fiend! Who made me so?" (p. 164)

Hester admits that she and Dimmesdale are responsible for what has become of Chillingworth, but her admission, elicited by the emotion of the moment, is incorrect. Chillingworth alone is responsible for his transformation. He has made himself a fiend by being unable to forgive the man who has wronged him. It is this vengeful inability to forgive and the consequences arising from it that remove Chillingworth from the human community and finally negate the small residue of sympathy that has been granted to him. It is also the inability to forgive and the revenge that it has generated that indict Chillingworth as the unpardonable sinner whose sin is far greater than the adultery of Hester and Dimmesdale.

Upon learning from Hester of the doctor's true identity, Dimmesdale himself passes the final judgment on Chillingworth and his activities: " 'I freely forgive you now [Hester]. May God forgive us both! We are not, Hester, the worst sinners in the world. There is one worse than even the polluted priest! That old man's revenge has been blacker than my sin. He has violated, in cold blood, the sanctity of the human heart. Thou and I, Hester, never did so!' " (p. 185)

Once aware of the evil machinations of his doctor-confidant, Dimmesdale is able to free himself from Chillingworth's grasp. In an inversion of the usual course of the doctor-patient relationship, the minister, able at last to confess his hidden and festering guilt, *cures himself* of his sickness, and in doing so is able to die in peace. Yet, ironically, Dimmesdale's confession and salvation come about precisely *because* Chillingworth has used his role as doctor in an attempt to sicken and destroy rather than heal the object of his revenge. Dimmesdale's dying words, uttered on the scaffold that is the only place where he can escape Chillingworth's malevolence, testify to the multiple ironies implicit in the relationship between the two men:

> "God knows; and he is merciful! He hath proved his mercy, most of all, in my afflictions. By giving me this burning torture to bear upon my breast! By sending yonder dark and terrible old man, to keep the torture always at red-heat! By bringing me hither, to die this death of triumphant ignominy before the people! Had either of these agonies been wanting, I had been lost for ever!" (p. 241)

Dimmesdale's salvation can only destroy Chillingworth whose black revenge is not only frustrated but, and still worse for the avenger, transformed into the unintended agent of his patient's cure. Thus the moral recovery of the patient leads directly to the destruction of the doctor in an appropriate resolution of their perverted relationship. Chillingworth, who had come to live only for revenge, can only die when that revenge is thwarted.

Within a year of Dimmesdale's death, Chillingworth also dies, a blasted and defeated man. In this defeat, brought about by the unwanted cure of his patient, Chillingworth is distinctly the doctor as arch-fiend and fellow-sinner along with Ethan Brand, Aylmer, and Rappaccini. Clearly though, Chillingworth's evil is greater than that of the others; they at least were motivated initially by less than base ends. Chillingworth, motivated solely by his desire to achieve revenge, is Hawthorne's most powerful symbol of the potential for evil that lies within all doctors (in fact, within all people) whose expertise and influence over the lives of those they serve leave them especially vulnerable to the withering effects of the baser portion of their selves.[12] Without the restraint that would have controlled his excesses, Chillingworth becomes the prototype of the negative and feared potentiality of the doctor as manipulator and ultimate destroyer. As such, he is the total antithesis of what people hoped their doctors were, as well as the polar opposite of the image of the doctor that would evolve in the literature of the ensuing decades.

HOLMES AND MITCHELL: DOCTORS OF GOOD CHARACTER

To move from Hawthorne's doctors to those of Oliver Wendell Holmes and S. Weir Mitchell is to move from darkness and fear to the beginnings of light and hope. Holmes and Mitchell, physicians and friends who both wrote their cumbersome and melodramatic novels avocationally, brought to their fiction an understanding of patients' needs coupled with their first-hand knowledge of what doctors in the last half of the nineteenth century actually could do. They also grounded their novels in their own beliefs about how doctors should behave in their relations with patients. Spanning the closing decades of the nineteenth century, the medical novels of these two physician-writers presented fictional doctors far different from Hawthorne's Unpardonable Sinners. The doctors of Holmes and Mitchell are, on the whole, benevolent and wise men, able to soothe though seldom to cure body and spirit. Their limited abilities and their good character and gentle bedside manner combine to establish a portrait of the doctor that is strikingly different from that presented in Hawthorne's fiction. In the place of misdirected genius and malevolence that strive for perverted goals and in so doing wreak destruction, there is now benevolent care that soothes and aids, even while it fails to attain fully its own desired goal of curing. These doctors, the fictional counterparts of what American physicians in the post-Civil War decades were striving to become, are the very embodiment of upright character and proper behavior. Holmes's first medical novel, *Elsie Venner* (1859) is subtitled *A Romance of Destiny*, and in the Preface to the first edition, Holmes explains that he chose to call his narrative a "romance" in order "to make sure of being indulged in the common privileges of the poetic license."[13] What he most requires indulgence in are the fantastical elements that tax a reader's belief that the novel's title character could have been so thoroughly influenced in both her appearance and behavior by the prenatal snakebite that affected her, allegedly, for life.

Although Elsie Venner is the central character, Holmes does more than merely present a case study in the unraveling of prenatal influences. He uses Elsie's snakelike characteristics to explore the underlying question of the limits of individual moral responsibility, the theological issue that undergirds all three of his medical novels. As the case study and the theological debate unfold, the New England social world in which Elsie Venner lives and dies is presented in a leisurely and detailed way that grounds the more fantastic elements of the tale in a commonplace reality and establishes the credibility of the narrator, who is the first of the three doctors presented in the novel.

Both as a characterizing device and as a means to make the novel's more romantic and allegorical elements acceptable to a reader, the narrative strategy is noteworthy. The story of Elsie Venner is told by a professor of medicine whose prize student, Bernard Langdon, takes a leave of absence from his studies to earn needed money. Langdon goes as a schoolteacher to the town of Rockland where he meets the other main characters, including Elsie Venner and her trusted physician, the elderly Dr. Kittredge. This narrative framework allows Holmes to present three very different types of doctors: the professor, the bright and promising doctor-in-training, and the wise old general practitioner. What emerges from this composite is a view of the limits of the medical profession in the midnineteenth century as well as a clear depiction of how crucial a doctor's character and behavior are to the good that he is able to achieve, in spite of his professional limitations.

The professor of medicine remains in the background, appearing only seldom in the story he relates, and Bernard Langdon functions almost exclusively as a teacher rather than as a medical student. Most prominent and at the tale's moral center is the normative figure, Dr. Kittredge. For all of his importance, though, Kittredge does not appear until almost a full hundred pages have elapsed. The delay in his introduction is characteristic of the novel's slowly unwinding plot. Before meeting Kittredge, the reader is treated to a description of "The Brahmin Caste of New England," introduced to Bernard Langdon as he embarks on his stop-gap teaching career, and presented with an enigmatic first glimpse of Elsie Venner: " . . . a strange, wild-looking girl . . . winding a gold chain about her wrist, and then uncoiling it, as if in a kind of reverie" (p. 52).

This first mysterious introduction of Elsie Venner concludes the fourth chapter and is immediately followed by "An Old Fashioned Descriptive Chapter," in which the town of Rockland, its geography, architecture, churches, public houses, and schools are described at length. The pattern of rising suspense alternating with more commonplace description and action continues throughout the novel. In the sixth chapter, "The Sunbeam and the Shadow," Bernard Langdon's fellow-teacher, Helen Darley, is apprehensive about a composition "written in a singular, sharp-pointed, long slender hand, on a kind of wavy, ribbed paper . . . The subject of the paper was The Mountain,—the composition being a sort of descriptive rhapsody . . . As the teacher read on, her color changed, and a kind of tremulous agitation came over her." The agitation increases until she works herself into a nervous spasm.

Only after the paroxysm is over, in fact only after the narrator actually raises the question of the severity of the cause of the nervous attack by saying, "Perhaps it is of no great consequence what was in the composition which set her off," does the reader learn that the theme is "signed in the same peculiar, sharp, slender hand, *E. Venner*" (p. 72). This added bit of information about Elsie is set off against (if not altogether neutralized by) the professor-narrator's comment that Helen Darley "was in such a state that almost any slight agitation would have brought on the attack . . . that it was the accident of her transient excitability, very probably, which made a trifling cause the seeming occasion of so much disturbance" (p. 73). Here, in a manner akin to what Hawthorne does in "Rappaccini's Daughter," Holmes calls into question the validity of Helen Darley's response to Elsie Venner, and thereby forces the reader to suspend judgment about the mysterious girl.

This suspension is crucial to the novel's overall effect. Although Elsie does, in fact, behave in strange and sometimes dangerous ways, her behavior is not wholly her responsibility, and she cannot be judged evil for what she is and does. For Holmes, Elsie is much like Beatrice Rappaccini, a victim of external forces and thus not to be held responsible for her acts. This central issue of the limits of individual responsibility is spoken to directly by Holmes in his "Second Preface" to the novel, written in 1883: "Was Elsie Venner, poisoned by the venom of a crotalus before she was born, morally responsible for the 'volitional' abberations, which translated into acts become what is known as sin, and, it may be, what is punished as crime?" (p. x). Holmes argues that she is not responsible for the poisoning over which she had no control, and he extends his argument outward to include "the unfortunate victim who received a moral poison from a remote ancestor before he drew his first breath" (p. x). These are the crucial questions that the novel raises, and crucial to the reader's resolution of them is the good Dr. Kittredge, "the leading physician of Rockland . . . a shrewd old man, who looked pretty keenly into his patients through his spectacles, and pretty widely at men, women, and things in general over them" (p. 98). Once introduced, Kittredge is never far from the center of things, and the image of him as the keen, careful observer continues throughout the novel. Meeting Elsie who has come, unexpectedly, to a large party, Kittredge chats with the girl: "The doctor laughed good-naturedly, as if this were an amusing bit of pleasantry,—but he lifted his head and dropped his eyes a little, so as to see her through his spectacles" (p. 100). Kittredge's observations of Elsie made over many years are as astute in their way as are those made by Ethan Brand in his quest for the Unpardonable Sinner. Yet there is a singular and vital difference. Brand had studied his subjects in order to manipulate them to his own ends; Kittredge studies Elsie in order to know better how to treat her and how to advise her father about her care. The knowledge that a doctor comes necessarily to have of a patient, knowledge fraught with implicit danger in Hawthorne's fiction, is being used for far different ends in the fiction of Holmes.

Because Kittredge has come to know Elsie so well, he functions as the primary vehicle for explaining her to her father, Dudley Venner, to Bernard Langdon, to the people of Rockland, and indirectly to the reader. Kittredge has argued against sending Elsie to an asylum and has advised, instead, that the willful and unmanageable girl be given as much freedom as possible and watched with care and discretion (p. 147). As advisor to Dudley Venner, Kittredge provides "dry, hard advice . . . given from a kind heart, with a moist eye, and in tones which tried to be cheerful and were full of sympathy" (p. 195). Not only does he advise her father, but he also comes as near as possible to being a friend to Elsie; he encourages "all her harmless fancies . . . rarely reminding her that he was a professional advisor, except when she came out of her own accord, as in the talk they had at the party, telling him of some wild trick she had been playing" (p. 196).

Just as Kittredge serves as Elsie's mentor, so does he become the advisor to Bernard Langdon. At their first lengthy encouter, Langdon asks if the old doctor has an "extensive collection of medical works"; Kittredge's response quickly establishes him as a doctor who values experience more than he values formal education and scientific medicine.

> "Why, no," said the old Doctor, "I haven't got a great many printed books; and what I have I don't read quite as often as I might, . . . I'll tell you though, Mr. Langdon, when a man that's once started right lives among sick folks for five-and-thirty years, as I've done, if he hasn't got a library of five-and-thirty volumes bound up in his head at the end of that time, he'd better stop driving round and sell his horse and sulky. . . . I don't want to undervalue your science . . . but I know these people about here . . . so as all the science in the world can't know them, without it takes time about it, and sees them grow up and grow old, and how the wear and tear of life comes to them. You can't tell a horse by driving him once . . . nor a patient by talking half an hour with him."
> (pp. 210–11)

In contrast to the nonscientific, experiential approach of the old-fashioned doctor, Holmes juxtaposes his narrator, the professor of medicine, as spokesman for a more scientific and book-oriented mode of diagnosis and treatment. Having learned what he can from Dr. Kittredge about Elsie Venner's strange behavior, the still-puzzled Langdon writes to his professor about the possibility of ophidian influences and also about the question of inherited predispositions. The correspondence between the two comprises the bulk of chapter sixteen ("Epistolary"), and it is clear from the professor's response that he is a far different kind of doctor from the old-fashioned Kittredge. To answer Langdon, the professor looks "into the old books— into Schenckius and Turner and Kenelm Digby and the rest," and he turns to the "old authors . . . Actius and Paulus, both men of authority" as well as "to Andreas Baccius and Gaffarel" (pp. 220–22).

The professor concludes his weighty discourse to Langdon by giving an atypically straightforward piece of advice: *"Treat bad men as if they were insane.* They are *in-sane*, out of health, morally" (p. 228). Here Holmes allows the professor's ideas to come close to those of Kittredge, who later in the book echoes these very sentiments, saying (in a chapter-long argument with Reverend Doctor Honeywood about the differences between doctors and ministers) that where "we [doctors] are constantly seeing weakness . . . you [clergymen] see depravity" (p. 323). Yet in spite of their philosophical agreement, the professor among his books is able only to comment on and record the activities of those involved with Elsie, whereas Kittredge, the busy general practitioner, is the one who acts and gives care and sound advice. The advice that Kittredge gives Langdon about how to keep his eyes open and his heart shut lest he come, disastrously, to love Elsie Venner, serves in time to save the young man's life. The doctor knows that Langdon is in danger from Elsie's cousin, Dick Venner, who sees her infatuation with her schoolmaster as a threat to his own scheme to marry her and to inherit her father's estate. Holmes uses this melodramatic subplot to characterize Kittredge further by showing him to be both clever and protective as well as benevolent; in good time, the doctor's careful observations and wise counsel enable Langdon to survive Dick Venner's murderous assault (pp. 369–74).

Kittredge's compassion and wisdom, evident in his attitude and behavior toward Elsie and Langdon, are also apparent as the doctor talks with another of his patients, Reverend Mr. Fairweather, about the attempt on Langdon's life. Here again, the humane kindness of the doctor is juxtaposed to the more severe and judgmental responses of the clergyman. Fairweather condemns Dick Venner's action and asserts that his soul is lost. In response, the doctor claims that the young man " 'has some humanity left in him yet' " and goes on to say, " 'I can't judge men's souls ... I can judge their acts, and hold them responsible for those,—but I don't know much about their souls. If you or I had found our soul in a half-breed body [like Dick Venner's], and been turned loose to run among the Indians, we might have been playing just such tricks as this fellow had been trying. What if you or I had inherited all the tendencies that were born with his cousin Elsie?' " (pp. 402–3).

At this point, Holmes is giving Kittredge the advantage in the novel's central debate about the limits of individual responsibility. The doctor continues to appear thoroughly admirable as the compassionate and wise man dealing with the weak and foolish minister. Fairweather has long suffered from his growing desire to leave his own troublesome pulpit and join the far more, for him, soothing Catholic Church, and he has come to consult Kittredge about more than mere physical discomfort. The troubled minister is in search of advice. As the doctor and the minister talk, Holmes describes the encounter in a way that echoes Hawthorne's description of Chillingworth's fiendish pursuit of Arthur Dimmesdale's hidden sin. As Kittredge tells Fairweather not to remain " 'in the wrong pulpit,' " the clergyman feels considerable relief. "The Reverend Mr. Fairweather breathed with more freedom. The Doctor saw into his soul through those awful spectacles of his,—into and beyond, as one sees through a thin fog. But it was with a real human kindness, after all" (p. 405). Again, Holmes affirms the positive value and the necessity of a doctor's coming to know a patient thoroughly and intimately in order to be able to provide aid and comfort. This complete knowledge, though, must be gained with "real human kindness" if the doctor is to avoid the risk of exploiting or harming the patient about whom so much is known.

Holmes also makes clear that it is far more effective for a doctor to be able to look into a patient's soul, as Kittredge does, than it is to look only into the old books as the scholarly professor admits to doing. It is Kittredge with his intimate firsthand knowledge and insight who is held up as the ideal doctor, far more worthy of emulation than the others presented in the novel. Yet when presented with a true challenge to his expertise, even the ideal physician reaches the limit of his abilities. Though Kittredge can advise and soothe Elsie, he cannot finally cure her because her malady transcends his limited medical powers.

As death approaches, Elsie becomes more and more humanized as she is freed from the snakelike portion of herself. As her strength wanes, she becomes more her untainted self, and Kittredge is less able to help her. "Her heart beat more feebly every day,—so that the old doctor himself, with all his experience, could see nothing to account for the gradual failing of the powers of life, and yet could find no remedy which seemed to arrest its progress in the smallest degree" (p. 453).

In contrast to his detailed treatment of Kittredge, Holmes pays considerably less attention to the doctors in his other medical novels, *The Guardian Angel* (1867)[14] and *A Mortal Antipathy* (1885)[15]. However, even though they are minor characters, these physicians are portrayed in much the same positive light that Holmes focuses on the good Dr. Kittredge. In both novels as in *Elsie Venner*, Holmes distinguishes clearly between what his doctors actually can do to cure and how they should and how they do behave as they tend their patients. This divided emphasis lets the reader recognize the limits of the doctor's expertise in the decades when Holmes wrote; at the same time it continues to assert that all doctors, in their relations with patients, should emulate the kind of model practitioner that Kittredge was, regardless of his limitations. Holmes's doctors do not have the power that was evident in Hawthorne's physician-scientists. What his doctors do have, though, and what is power enough for their time are good sense, benevolent intentions, a clear and careful eye, and the genuine and earned trust of their patients. Holmes's main concern is not with the doctor as a professional with great expertise, but with the doctor as a person who should behave in very particular ways in the doctor-patient relationship. Holmes does not idealize his own fictional doctors in terms of power or expertise; that idealization could not occur until the actuality of the medical profession allowed such a shift in emphasis and portrayal. For Holmes, unlike Hawthorne, character and good sense, not skill and power are the crucial determinants of a doctor's goodness and usefulness. They are the traits to be expected by patients and emulated by their doctors.

Much the same thing is true in the medical fiction of S. Weir Mitchell, well-known physician and friend of Holmes. Mitchell's fiction spans the end of the nineteenth and the beginning of the twentieth centuries, as the American medical profession was just beginning to develop a new base of knowledge for its practice, police its own ranks, consolidate its power, and gain the public's trust. His fiction presents readers with a collection of doctors more varied in type than those of Holmes but equally limited in what they could do to cure their patients. Mitchell's doctors, as do Holmes's, further demonstrate the crucial importance of character and appropriate behavior as the primary determinants of their effectiveness and worth.

Mitchell deals with the effects of a doctor's flawed character in his first full-length novel, *In War Time* (1885). The inversion of the ideal image that Mitchell had presented in an earlier short story about the quack Ezra Sandcraft is used at greater length and with more subtlety in the presentation of Dr. Ezra Wendell, whose character flaws undermine and eventually destroy his potential for good. From the start, Ezra Wendell is portrayed as a weak man, temperamentally unsuited for the demands of medicine. Wendell is a "contract-assistant surgeon ... taken from civilian life and paid at a certain rate per month to do the duty of a military surgeon."[16] Once this fact is established, Mitchell's narrator notes that among these contract surgeons could be found both the most able men in the profession as well as those less competent who were happy to receive their monthly stipend of $ 80. The narrator continues with a sentence that characterizes the essence of Wendell and is a foreshadowing of the downward course that his career will take throughout the novel: "Among these latter were many of those hapless persons who drift through life, and seize, as they are carried along, such morsels of good luck as the great tides of fortune float within reach of their feeble tentacula" (p. 3).

That Wendell is one of these "hapless persons" is well established early in the novel, whose plot chronicles his downfall and its effect on others. "A man of full middle height," who is slightly stooped, Wendell's features are "distinct but delicate" with a "mouth ... too regular for manly beauty." To the eyes of others, he presents both an "interesting face" and a "careless figure." That he is the antithesis of the stalwart physician is readily apparent from his "certain look of indifference to appearances," an indifference that leads him to carry a sun umbrella "at a lazy slope over the shoulder" (pp. 3, 4).

Enriching the emerging portrait is Wendell's sister, Ann, who accompanies him to the military hospital and who is concerned with his sloppiness and his continual tardiness. Declining his offer to relieve her of a basket of supplies that she has been carrying, she indicates that she is well accustomed to carrying many of his burdens: " 'It is not heavy ... and I am well used to it. But I do think, brother Ezra, we must hurry. Why cannot you hurry! You are half an hour late, and do look at your vest! It is buttoned all crooked ... ' " (p. 5).

Once arrived at the military hospital, Wendell, irritated by being reprimanded for his tardiness, turns moody and displays more of his flawed character:

> He was one of those unhappy people who are made sore for days by petty annoyances; nor did the possession of considerable intelligence and much imagination help him. In fact, these qualities served only, as is usual in such

natures, to afford him a more ample fund of self-torment. In measuring himself with others, he saw that in acquisitions and mind he was their superior, and he was constantly puzzled to know why he failed where they succeeded (pp. 8,9).

The reasons for Wendell's failure soon become evident. About to leave the hospital for the day, he is interrupted and told about the death of one of his patients; he feels "vaguely that his own mood had prevented him from giving the young man such efficient advice as might have made him more careful. The thought was not altogether agreeable" (p. 17). Further emphasizing his weak character is the ease with which Wendell rationalizes his questionable conduct:

> He soon reasoned himself into his usual state of self-satisfied calm. It was after all a piece of bad fortune, and attended with no consequences to himself; one of many deaths, the every day incidents of a raging war and of hospital life. Very likely it would have happened soon or late, let him have done as he might. A less imaginative man would have suffered less; a man with more conscience would have suffered longer, and been the better for it. (p. 18)

That Wendell suffers neither much nor long is evident on his walk home-ward as he drops and shatters his meerschaum pipe and has "a shock of sudden misery, as he [sees] it by the moonlight in fragments; a shock which, as he reflected a moment later, seemed to him—nay, which was—quite as great as that caused by the death of his patient, an hour before!" (p. 18).

One final touch is added to this early indictment of Wendell as he is in his study, sketching "with much adroitness" what he is observing through his microscope. Here in a scene that might belie some of what has already been shown of Wendell's weak nature, the narrator takes care to comment: "It is possible for some men to pursue every object, their duties and their pleasures, with equal energy, nor is it always true that the Jack-of-all-trades is master of none; but it was true of this man that, however well he did things,—and he did many things well,—he did none with sufficient intensity of purpose, or with such steadfastness of effort as to win high success in any one of them" (pp. 28–29).

The broad outlines of Wendell's character are established by the end of the second chapter. In the remainder of the novel, Mitchell presents that character in action and continuously delineates a standard of right behavior against which Wendell, the man who lacks *sufficient intensity of purpose*, is measured:

> He did his work, and, as he was intelligent, often did it well; but his medical conscience, overweighted by the need for incessant wakefulness, and enfeebled by natural love of ease and of mere intellectual luxuries, suffered from the

life he led, and carried into his after days more or less of the resultant evil. Happily for his peace of mind as for that of many doctors, no keen critic followed him, or could follow him, through the little errors of unthoughtful work, often great in result, which grew as he continued to do his slipshod tasks. Like all men who practice that which is part art, part science, he lived in a world of possible, and I may say reasonable, excuses for failures; and no man knew better than he how to use his intellect to apologize to himself for lack of strict obedience to the moral code by which his profession justly tests the character of its own labor. (p. 45)

By the novel's end, it is Wendell's repeated violation of his profession's moral code that brings about his downfall and enables Mitchell to show how a doctor should *not* behave. When asked to continue caring for Major Morton, who had been his patient in the military hospital, Wendell is pleased because his own superficial gentility is flattered, and he looks forward to the wealthy atmosphere of the Morton's household and circle of friends. In describing Wendell's clear preference for wealthy patients, the narrator softens neither the description nor the judgment of Wendell's attitude toward those patients with little or no money:

The poor whom he attended he did not like... Indeed, he disliked all that belonged to poverty, as he did other unpleasing things. He saw this class of patients knowing that he must, but made brief visits, and found true interest impossible where his senses and taste were steadily in revolt. Perhaps as a doctor of the rich alone he might have done better. It seems probable that he should never have been a doctor at all. (p. 63)

In this explicit comment, Mitchell provides a summary of the rest of the novel during which Wendell shows again and again, through increasingly serious breaches of conduct, his unsuitability for his profession.

How it is possible for Wendell to succeed, even minimally, in spite of his weak character and professional limitations is largely explained in a passage that has the narrator addressing the question of the disparity between the reality and appearance of Ezra Wendell who has just come upon a new idea for a research project. He is elated because he can now set aside other of his research that has reached the point where he cannot go on with it. In explaining Wendell's limitations as a researcher, the narrator details how very differently a doctor of Wendell's sort can appear to the various groups who know him:

In fact, his mental ambitions were high, his power to pursue them limited; while his capacity to be pleased with the recurrent dreams of possible future intellectual achievements was as remarkable as his failure to see why he constantly failed to realize them. Hence, while respected as a man with much general and scientific knowledge, he was known among doctors as having contributed nothing to their journals save barren reports of cases, and to naturalists as a clear amateur. But of these siftings of a man by his fellows, the public which is to use him learns little or nothing, so that...[to patients] he represented the brilliant and original physician, to be justified by the patient issues of the years which go to the slow growth of a doctor's reputation. (pp. 198–99)

Wendell's reputation, even though aided by his sister's work and attention and bolstered by the patronage of the Mortons and their friends, is unable to withstand the undermining influence of his own weak character. The reality of Ezra Wendell comes to overtake the appearance that he projects and signals the start of his decline. In the course of that decline, Mitchell takes care to explain and to show that without the requisite character traits, no one, no matter how clever or charming, can hope to succeed as a doctor.

The decline in Wendell's professional fortunes is detailed closely, and it is easy to see that Mitchell intends to talk of more than just a single fictional character. Wendell's weaknesses would undermine the work and effectiveness of any doctor. Recommended by the Mortons, Wendell had gained access to numerous wealthy patients, willing to consult him on a trial basis.

As time went on he lost a larger proportion of such patients than he should have done. He was in every way an agreeable and amusing visitor, but when he had to sustain the courage of the sick and satisfy watchful friends through grave illnesses he failed. For some reason, he did not carry confidence to others; perhaps because he was unable to hide his mental unstableness, which showed in too frequent changes of opinion. Moreover, his love of ease made impossible for him the never-ending daily abandonment of this moment of quiet, or that litttle bit of tranquil home life, which every wise physician counts upon once for all as part of the discomforts which he must accept if he means to win success. (pp. 234–35)

Fundamentally lazy, unwilling to accept discomfort, unable to trust himself enough to be able to engender confidence in his patients, concerned more with his own ease than with his patients' needs, Wendell is the antithesis of the benevolent, effective, and caring doctor. How far he deviates from the implicit norm against which he is compared is abundantly clear by the novel's end. In a characteristic moment of carelessness, Wendell makes a medication error that is lethal to young Edward Morton, and in a panic he connives to shift the blame to his victim's brother. Succeeding with his deception, he further compounds his duplicity by accepting an indirect bribe from the dead man's mother, who believes that Wendell has protected her surviving son's reputation when in fact he has protected only himself. Soon, though, the full truth emerges, Wendell confesses, and he is fully revealed as the weak and flawed man he has always been.

Once Wendell has confessed, the novel moves rapidly to its close. The last information about Wendell is that he has gone off to the West for a "fresh start," but any sense of hope or self-improvement in this move is quickly undercut. In the concluding pages, Mrs. Morton receives a letter from Ann Wendell who tells the full truth about her brother's responsibility for Edward Morton's death and concludes by saying that Wendell is "much broken in health and spirit." What little sympathy might be aroused by this information is dampened by the narrator's final comment: "When Alice saw this note, a good while after it was written, she had a great longing to be able to say some tender words to the true, simple, honest woman, who had poured out the waters of her loving life where the barren soil seemed to give back no least return" (p. 423).

Though harsh, this final reference to Wendell as "barren soil" is appropriate, given the downward spiral of his life and career. What little he achieves as a doctor is totally overshadowed by the weak and selfish character that Mitchell goes to such lengths to establish. In that flawed character and in the consequences attendant upon it are visible the dangers and the problems that arise when a person temperamentally unsuited and lacking sufficient intensity of purpose mistakenly embarks upon a medical career. Mitchell, in his portrait of the barren Ezra Wendell, shows by inversion much the same thing that Holmes had shown by more direct and positive portrayal: the value and usefulness of a doctor depend not only on expertise and power but also on the goodness and appropriateness of character in its several manifestations.

In striking contrast to Ezra Wendell is Owen North, physician and raconteur, who is the first-person narrator of Mitchell's two "conversation novels," *Characteristics* (1891) and its sequel, *Dr. North and His Friends* (1900). These two books, written initially for serial publication in *The Century*, continue to exhibit Mitchell's concern with the doctor's proper character, but in them character is revealed almost exclusively through talk rather than through action. Rambling, overblown, and at times tedious, the books are nevertheless of interest here because they vary Mitchell's usual presentation of the doctor in action while extending the ideal image of the admirable doctor of good character by means of Owen North's leisurely talk about himself, his friends, and his profession.

At the start of *Characteristics*, Dr. North takes care to establish the selfless and altruistic nature of his entry into medicine, saying that he took to it out of interest rather than necessity, since at the age of twenty-one he was a "man of ample means, free to do as [he] liked."[17] His altruism is further exhibited by his volunteering to put his surgical skills to work in support of the Union Army. Shot in the spine and paralyzed, North has the opportunity to turn his doctor's keen eye on the bedside manners of those doctors who attend his case. Pointing out that "the sick man is a shrewd detective, and soon or late gets at the true man inside of the doctor" (p. 7), North goes on to describe various doctors' bedside manners.

He expresses dismay at "men who possess cheap manufactured manners adapted, as they believe, to the wants of the 'sick-room'—a term [he] loathe[s]." Next he praises "the rarer man who is naturally tender in his contact with the sick, and who is by good fortune full of educated tact. He has the dramatic quality of instinctive sympathy, and above all, knows how to control it. If he has directness of character, too, although he may make mistakes (as who does not?), he will be, on the whole, the best advisor for the sick" (pp. 7, 8).

Having described the worst and the best kinds of bedside manners, North adds a comment that indicates that there is still something beyond rational explanation in the character of those doctors who are most soothing to their patients:

> "But over and above all this there is, as I have urged, some mystery in the way in which certain men refresh the patient with their presence. I fancy that every doctor who has this power—and sooner or later he is sure to know that he has it—also learns that there are days when he has it not. It is in part a question of his own physical state; at times the virtue has gone out of him."
> (p. 8)

The mystery that North mentions adds an element of the near-magical to the more pedestrian qualities already established as necessary for the admirable and beneficient doctor to possess.

Later, North comes to a more direct presentation of himself as a doctor, after agreeing to take a curious friend along for a tour of the hospital. The stage is set here for a chapter-long description of North, the capable doctor, thoroughly in control of the people and situations he encounters. North's control and the orderliness of his professional life (exaggerated as they are) find an echo in his description of the exaggeratedly clean hospital ward through which he guides his friend:

> The walls, like the floors, were of exquisite cleanliness, and unornamented save by portraits of physicians who had gone their rounds for years in these wards, and at last followed their many patients out of this world...
> Here were some twenty beds, all full. Beside each was a little table, and now, neatly tucked back, clean fly-nets, it being near to summer. The floor was of spotless boards; the walls were of a pleasant gray tone, and there was ample light, and, of course, abundant air, so that the atmosphere was without odor. (p. 53)

The neat, spotless, and odorless hospital ward is an appropriate setting for North, the ideal physician for whom order and control are normative, and death the ultimate enemy. When asked by his friend about the sadness of the medical profession, North answers that death per se does not sadden him because it is an "ever-repeated" inevitability. Then, in words strangely reminiscent of the malevolent Rappaccini, he acknowledges his allegiance to the unattainable ideal of his profession: "What I personally hate is defeat, by death, by incurable ailments. I have the feeling which all physicians ought to have that every one should get well; that all disease is curable somehow. It is, I suspect, the intellectual defeat I so dislike; but there is a host of compensations' " (pp. 61–62).

Among these compensations is the beneficial effect of a medical career on the character of the individual doctor, a compensation that North elaborates on during a conversation about the influence of work on character. His words, cool and detached, bring to mind the decline of Ezra Wendell. North says:

> "Every occupation has its influence on character, be that what it may. My own profession is full of temptations to yield to little meannesses. It is a constant trial of temper. It offers ample chance to win in retail ways by disparagement of others, and by flattery and appearance of interest where little is felt. The small man—what I may call the retail nature—gives way to these temptations; the nobler nature strengthens in resisting them. A doctor's lifework is the best education for the best characters. It is the worst for the small of soul." (pp. 161–62)

Using North as his spokesman, Mitchell is summarizing here the bulk of his fiction in its concern for the primacy of character and the effects of a medical career on people of varying sorts.

Having established the good and appropriate character of Owen North, Mitchell goes on in *Dr. North and His Friends* to demonstrate and embellish it further. The second of the conversation novels begins five years after North's marriage, and it is even more rambling and tedious than its predecessor. As in *Characteristics*, the format of *Dr. North and His Friends* consists of the continual gathering together, at meals, at teas, at parties, and so on, of the doctor's numerous friends who talk, trade anecdotes, share gossip, and characterize themselves and each other through their chatter. At the center of this witty though brittle circle stands Owen North, narrating, participating, commenting, and exhibiting throughout the character and control that Mitchell has established for the successful doctor.

Another trait of the successful doctor is presented as North talks of the need for the healer to accept the mystery of things:

> "The physician is credited with want of faith in things spiritual. The charge is common and has classical support, and yet of all people he is the one most often called upon to think and act with decision in cases where action must rest on incomplete knowledge. He moves amid mystery. If he does not intellectually respect the complex riddles of soul, mind, and body, and their interdependence, he is unfit for the higher seats in the temple of the god of medicine."[18]

Continuing his discussion of intuitive diagnosis, North speaks directly to the complex skill of careful and accurate assessment and admits that he acts, everyday, " 'on beliefs which no man could entirely justify by proof.' " Then he says:

> I must put my conclusion on ground where Clayborne and others could stand with me. This is a common experience with the best of my guild. It is the power to reason from uncertain premises to conclusions as often unsure that makes the best physician. He practices an art not yet a science. It is based on many sciences. A man may know them all and be a less skillful healer than one who, knowing them less well, is master of the art to which they increasingly contribute." (p. 457)

Here, North articulates yet again the importance of right character, an importance so great that it can actually go beyond mere learning in terms of what it enables a doctor to do. Having spoken as diagnostician and believer in the art rather than just the science of medicine, North goes on to conclude his rambling novel by describing the foreign travels, talks, and intrigues of his friends. Rather than ending with any sense of finality, the book just winds down and stops. Ending as abruptly as it began, the second of Mitchell's conversation novels adds little new to the portrait of Dr. Owen North already established in *Characteristics*; what the sequel does provide is further occasion for the wise and benevolent doctor to demonstrate his character largely in nonmedical situations through his talk with and observations about his friends and colleagues.

The indirect characterization that Mitchell uses to present Owen North is abandoned for a more direct and effective portrayal of the ideal doctor in action in *Circumstance* (1901); more a social than a medical novel, its story of the rise and fall of the fortune-hunting Lucretia Hunter occupies the bulk of Mitchell's concern. However, standing at the center of the novel's social world and functioning as Mrs. Hunter's wise and observant adversary is Dr. Sidney Archer, another of Mitchell's doctors of good character. Though only occasional, there are pointed descriptions of Archer that both echo and extend the characterization of the "good doctor" established in Mitchell's earlier fiction. At the start of a visit to a patient, the elderly and wealthy John Fairthorne, Archer speaks to Fairthorne's niece about the need to minister to the total personality of a patient, not just to a specific ill, saying, " 'If one could go from bed to bed, and simply be the technical engineer of human machines, it would be easy; but these machines have mothers, and wives, and notions. One has to listen and prescribe for anxieties, and splint broken hopes.' "[19] Once finished tending Fairthorne, a patient for whom little can be done, Archer goes on to his next appointment, and the narrator provides a brief but laudatory description of him. "He was driven to his out-patient clinic, and gave himself head and heart to a business which requires ideal patience, perfect sweetness of character, and sympathetic insight" (p. 52).

In direct contrast to Archer is Dr. Thomas Soper, the incompetent doctor who knows little and does less. In Soper, Mitchell creates the perfect foil to Archer, and there is little time lost in establishing Soper's character with all of its deficiencies. The first description of Soper is a preview of all that will be seen of him: "Thomas Soper, M.D., was also LL.D. of some remote little Western college whose president he had once attended when that official was taken ill in the city. The doctor was a childless widower of advanced middle-age, described by mothers as a safe physician and by himself as a man who kept up to the times but never tried experiments. Sidney Archer said he never did anything else" (p. 232).

Throughout the novel, Mitchell does little more than tell about Archer as the admirable doctor, the antithesis of Dr. Soper, and there are markedly few occasions of Archer in any active role. The last one is a conversation with Martin Blount, his medical student assistant; Archer praises Blount's laboratory work and speaks of the art and science of medicine in a manner reminiscent of Dr. North.

> "Sit down, Blount, [Archer] said; "you are doing my work very well. There is nothing like the laboratory to train a man to exactness. Individuality must always keep our work at the bedside more or less an art. It never can have the precision of science so long as one man differs from another. So long as men differ there will be the chance of our being unable to forsee results with certainty.' " (p. 396)

Here, again, Mitchell has Archer speak indirectly of the importance of good and appropriate character, the very traits that allow a doctor to know and deal effectively with the individual differences of patients. In the particular case of Archer's care of John Fairthorne, the old man's eccentricities and his capricious dismissal of Archer make it impossible for the good doctor to save him. The old man's death, caused by a heart attack, in no way casts doubt on Archer's competence or goodness; to the reader's mind, Archer has done all that he can. He remains to the end the ideal personified in spite of the fact that in the course of the novel he does very little actual doctoring. This lack of active care is consistent with Mitchell's emphasis on the character rather than on the expertise and the action of his fictional doctors. Archer, as Owen North and as Holmes's fictional doctors, is admirable and worthy of emulation far less for what he accomplishes than for the kind of person he is.

HOWELLS AND JEWETT: OF WOMEN DOCTORS WEAK AND STRONG

The concern of both Holmes and Mitchell with the importance of proper character in determining a doctor's worth and effectiveness is echoed with notable variations in the medical novels of William Dean Howells and Sarah Orne Jewett, who focus their attention on the struggles of women doctors to break through the barriers between them and their chosen career. Although portraying two very different women in substantially different circumstances, both Howells and Jewett emphasize the importance of character in the making of the ideally successful woman doctor. Even though both novelists focus their attention on young women fighting for a place in a male-dominated profession, there are—very much in evidence and crucial to the action of the two novels—men doctors, staunch and ever in control, much akin to those created by Holmes and Mitchell.

The presence of these normative male physicians is expectable and functionally useful for the fictional worlds being created. It is against these men that these women physicians will be judged and found either adequate or wanting by a reader more accustomed to a male-dominated medical world. Howells may describe his young woman doctor as acting "manishly" and Jewett may give her heroine, Nan Prince, a manly surname, but both women, though very different in character and ability and eventual success, must face and deal with the stultifying cultural burden imposed on all women who presume to enter a heretofore exclusively male domain. The markedly different ways in which these two women physicians are presented exemplify two extremes on the spectrum of responses to women who would attempt to enter medicine (and other professions) throughout the coming century.

Grace Breen, the title character of Howell's *Dr. Breen's Practice* (1881), is almost as unsuited for medicine as is Mitchell's Ezra Wendell. Part of Howell's ostensible purpose in the novel is to demonstrate that very unsuitability; furthermore, by establishing situations with which Dr. Breen cannot cope, Howells shows by inversion the traits that a successful doctor, woman or man, must possess. Grace Breen had decided, self-centeredly, to pursue a medical career after recovering from the pain of an unhappy love affair. Those who knew her well "understood that she had chosen this work with the intention of giving her life to it, in the spirit in which other women enter convents, or go out to heathen lands."[20] Burdened with a "New England girl's naturally morbid sense of duty," Breen, "rich enough to have no need of her profession as a means of support," embarks on a medical career with more thought to her own emotional needs than to the needs and problems of her future patients.

Following her graduation from the New York Homeopathic School, her initial plan is to return to her own town "and begin the practice of her profession among those who had always known her, and whose scrutiny and criticism would be hardest to bear, and therefore, as she fancied, the most useful in the formation of her character." This idea she gives up, however, and needing the help and support of a more experienced doctor, "she planned going to one of the great factory towns and beginning practice there, in the company with an older physician, among the children of the operatives." This plan is delayed, and while waiting to complete arrangements, Dr. Breen goes off with her mother to Jocelyn's, a New England seaside resort. Joining them unexpectedly is Grace Breen's old school friend, Louise Maynard, who "had arrived from the West, aimlessly sick and unfriended, just as they were about leaving home" (pp. 12,13).

In dealing with this unanticipated first patient, Dr. Breen discovers her limitations and confronts some of the obstacles that a woman doctor had to overcome in the late nineteenth century. Breen's greatest problem is her inability to transcend her own culturally induced sense of inferiority. She speaks cogently of this in a conversation with her mother:

> "I think it's rather hard, mother, that you be always talking as if I wished to take my calling manishly. All that I intend is not to take it womanishly; but as for not being a woman about it, or anything else, that's simply impossible. A woman is reminded of her insufficiency to herself every hour of the day. And it's always a man that comes to her help." (pp. 43–44)

Having spoken of a woman's "insufficiency to herself," Breen goes on to lament the problems that she (and other women choosing professional careers) face in the form of censure and distrust of other suspicious women. She says to her mother, " 'Oh, yes! Talk about men being obstacles! It's other women! There isn't a woman in the house that wouldn't sooner trust herself in the hands of the stupidest boy that got his diploma with me than she would in mine. Louise knows it, and she feels that she has a claim upon me in being my patient. And I've no influence with her about her conduct because she understands perfectly well that they all consider me much worse. She prides herself on doing me justice. She patronizes me. She tells me that I'm just as nice as if I hadn't been through all that' " (p. 44).

Yet, having been "through all that," having completed her training, Grace Breen still lacks self-confidence, one of the most crucial traits for a successful doctor. Unsure of her own expertise and functioning in a world that mistrusts her professional abilities because she is a woman, she has little chance to develop the strength of character she needs to succeed. That kind of strong character, however, is readily evident in the person of Dr. Rufus Mulbridge with whom Dr. Breen consults after Mrs. Maynard's condition worsens. Mulbridge, initially disconcerted and bemused to discover that the young woman who asks him to consult with her is, in fact, a doctor, does agree to see Mrs. Maynard, but upon learning that Dr. Breen is a homeopathist, he withdraws his assent with an embarrassed explanation that their professional differences make consultation impossible. Initially embarrassed and then angered by Mulbridge's refusal, Dr. Breen prepares to depart, but her lack of self-confidence and her fear for Mrs. Maynard's life combine to weaken her resolve. She agrees to turn the case over to Dr. Mulbridge, and she volunteers to help by taking on the task of nursing the patient.

Upon learning that her case is to be taken over by Mulbridge, Mrs. Maynard mounts, briefly, a show of protest that he would not consult with Dr. Breen. However, her anger and her loyalty to her friend fade rapidly: "It was her final resolution that when Dr. Mulbridge did come she would give him a piece of her mind; and she received him with anxious submissiveness, and hung upon all his looks and words with quaking and with an inclination to attribute her unfortunate symptoms to the treatment of her former physician" (pp. 106–7). This reversal of Mrs. Maynard's attitude is both a commentary on the capriciousness of patients as well as an indication that a patient's attitude is largely a result of the impression of competence and confidence generated by the doctor in charge. The impression that Mulbridge conveys as he examines Mrs. Maynard is seen through Grace Breen's eyes, but even allowing for the exaggeration resulting from her own lack of self-confidence, it is clear that Howells intends to represent the staunch, confident, and competent doctor, the proper foil to the improperly fearful Dr. Breen:

> Grace sat by and watched him with perfectly quiescent observance. The large, somewhat uncouth man gave evidence to her intelligence that he was all physician, and that he had not chosen his profession from any theory or motive, however good, but had been as much chosen by it as if he had been born a physcian. He was incredibly gentle and soft in all his movements, and perfectly kind, without being at any moment unprofitably sympathetic. He knew when to listen and when not to listen,—to learn everything from the quivering bundle of nerves before him without seeming to have learnt anything alarming; and he smiled when it would do her good to be laughed at, and treated her with such grave respect that she could not feel herself trifled with, nor remember afterwards any point of neglect. (p. 107)

The discrepancy between Mulbridge's confident "all physician" manner and Grace Breen's lack of confidence in both herself and in the capabilities of other women is evident in a brief interchange she has with Mr. Libby who has gone to send a telegram to Mrs. Maynard's husband. Learning that nearly all of the telegraph operators are women, Dr. Breen shows her surprise and her own distrust of women: " 'Oh!' She looked grave. 'Can they trust young girls with such important duties?' " (p. 111). Unaware that she has asked the very question that others have asked of her, Grace Breen demonstrates the extent to which she shares the bias against women functioning in nontraditional roles, the very bias she has already suffered from herself.

Within the context of the novel, gender issues exaggerate the point of what is right and beneficial in a doctor's character. For a profession only beginning (as medicine was in the 1890s) to establish its credibility in the public mind, the introduction of any kind of deviance within its ranks was a threat, and there could be nothing more deviant at the time than a woman doctor. The age-old priesthood of the male healer could little afford—or so it thought—to open its ranks to women, the subservient underclass that was only then, in the final quarter of the nineteenth century, beginning to demand entry into and equity within a heretofore all-male world. The dead weight of cultural restraints was virtually insurmountable. In Dr. Grace Breen, Howells chose to present a case study of a woman finally unable to break through these restraints.

Grace Breen's inability to transcend her socially constructed world becomes even more evident as Mrs. Maynard's pneumonia worsens. Dr. Mulbridge takes total charge of the case, usurping even the nursing function he had earlier allowed to Dr. Breen. He allows her to relieve him for only short periods of time, "but when he returned to his charge, he showed himself jealous of all that Grace had done involving the exercise of more than a servile discretion. When she asked him once if there were nothing else she could do, he said, 'Yes, keep those women and children quiet,' in a tone that classified her with both" (p. 178). Having been demoted from doctor to nurse and then from nurse to nothing more than an obtrusive and annoying bystander, Grace Breen finally retains not even the courage to ask Mulbridge about the course of Mrs. Maynard's recovery. In sharp contrast to the unsure and fearful young woman doctor is the idealized view of Dr. Mulbridge as he cares for the worsening Mrs. Maynard: "Dr. Mulbridge watched beside his patient, noting every change with a wary intelligence which no fact escaped and no anxiety clouded; alert, gentle, prompt; suffering no question, and absolutely silent as to all impressions" (p. 179).

No longer able to tolerate Mulbridge's silent condescension, Dr. Breen blurts out her demand that he tell her at once if Mrs. Maynard will live. Not at all ruffled by her distress and anger, Mulbridge responds in words that pinpoint the underlying character flaw from which Grace Breen suffers: " 'Dr. Breen,' he said, 'I saw a great deal of pneumonia in the army, and I don't remember a single case that was saved by the anxiety of the surgeon' " (p. 180). More than anything else, it is this anxiety, resulting from her diminished sense of self-worth and consequent lack of self-confidence, that makes Grace Breen an unsuitable doctor. Howells takes care to point out that the young woman also suffers from other liabilities that are antithetical to the necessary character of a useful, confidence-inspiring doctor. Mrs. Maynard, recovered and convalescing, gives Grace Breen advice that is pointed and sound:

> "You're not fit to be a doctor, Grace," she said. "You're too nervous and you're too conscientious. It isn't merely your want of experience. No matter how much experience you had, if you saw a case go wrong in your hands, you'd want to call in some one else to set it right. Do you suppose Dr. Mulbridge would have given me up to another doctor because he was afraid he couldn't cure me? No indeed! He'd have let me die first, and I shouldn't

have blamed him. Of course I know what pressure I brought to bear upon you, but you had no business to mind me. You oughtn't to have minded my talk any more than the buzzing of a mosquito and no real doctor would." (pp. 208–9)

Later on, while telling Dr. Mulbridge why she is giving up her medical career, Dr. Breen speaks more of the liabilities from which a woman doctor suffers, saying, " 'I believe that if Mrs. Maynard had had the same confidence in me that she would have had in any man I should not have failed. But every woman physician has a double disadvantage that I hadn't the strength to overcome,—her own inexperience and the distrust of other women' " (p. 221). The "double disadvantage" of which Grace Breen speaks is even more debilitating than she realizes. On one level, what she is able or unable to do has less to do with her training and ability than with the weakness and suitability of her character. More significantly, the defects of character— which Howells highlights in order to affirm the crucial role of right character in the making of a doctor—are greatly compounded by Grace Breen's being a woman. This compounding makes her task impossible. Had she been a man, her inappropriate character might yet have let her achieve her goal. Burdened with the added liability of being a woman who herself accepts society's belief that women are unable to do such things, she has no hope of success. As Grace Breen comes painfully to learn, to be a woman in pursuit of a career in medicine demands a character far more "right" than that demanded of any man.

This crucial role of right character is also the concern of Sarah Orne Jewett's first novel, *A Country Doctor* (1884). Herself the daughter of a physician, Jewett presents both the ideal general practitioner (the aging Dr. Leslie) and the young woman doctor-in-training (Nan Prince) whose character is strong enough for and appropriate to the arduous task she faces. The plot is simple. The orphaned Nan Prince, upon the death of her maternal grandmother, becomes the ward of Dr. Leslie, who rears her in a way that allows her to develop her natural capacities and interests without undue interference from society's gender-based constraints and expectations. Intent upon becoming a doctor, Nan Prince is encouraged and instructed by her guardian, but she meets considerable resistance from other segments of her world. Further complicating her life and weakening her resolve for a time is a romantic entanglement. However, the young woman endures the several tests of her dedication to medicine, reasserts her resolve, and goes on (unlike Grace Breen) to become the kind of ideal country doctor represented by her guardian.

Within this uncomplicated narrative structure, Jewett takes much care with her characterization of Dr. Leslie and Nan Prince, who together represent a complete expression of the medical idealization that was gaining strength in the closing decades of the century. From the start, Dr. Leslie is portrayed in glowing terms. He first appears to care for the dying Adeline Prince, mother of the baby girl who will later become his ward and assistant. Upon his arrival, he spreads comfort as only a loved and trusted country doctor can: "When he was fairly inside the Thacher kitchen, the benefaction of his presence was felt by everyone. It was most touching to see the patient's face lose its worried look, and grow quiet and comfortable as if here were some one on whom she could entirely depend.... There was something singularly self-reliant and composed about him; one felt that he was the wielder of great powers over the enemies, disease and pain, and that his brave hazel eyes showed a rare thoughtfulness and foresight."[21]

Beyond his thoughtfulness and foresight are other desirable attributes that go to make up the old country doctor's character. Foremost among these is his natural aptitude for medicine, spoken of directly by his old classmate and Navy surgeon, Dr. Ferris, who remarks on the difference between his own need to experiment and analyze in order to diagnose and Dr. Leslie's ability to reach an intuitive diagnosis: " 'You have the true gift for doctoring, you need no medical dictator, and whatever you study and whatever comes to you in the way of instruction simply ministers to your intuition. It grows to be a wonderful second-sight in a man such as you' " (p. 108).

The good doctor's second sight and his intuitive ability to diagnose are complemented by his compassion and humane concern for others, crucial attributes that are apparent in his affection for and rearing of Nan Prince. It is through the influence that he has upon his ward that Dr. Leslie is most fully characterized and implicitly praised. A fine doctor himself, he does the most difficult and important of things in transmitting his own knowledge, sensitivity, and concern to his protege.

Soon after going to live with Dr. Leslie, the young girl "might be seen every day by the doctor's side, as if he could not make his morning rounds without her...sitting soberly by when he dealt his medicines and gave advice, listening to his wise and merry talk with some and his helpful advice and consolation to others of the country people" (pp. 85–86). This early experience prompts her declaration that she " 'should best like to be a doctor' " (p. 86), a declaration that Dr. Leslie accepts with the realization that her welfare and the success of her dream depend greatly on the decisions he makes regarding her upbringing.

The nature of this upbringing is summarized as Dr. Leslie tells his old friend, Dr. Ferris, of the young girl's life: " 'There is one thing quite re-markable. I believe that she has grown up as naturally as a plant grows, not having been clipped back or forced in any unnatural direction. If ever a human being were untrammeled and left alone to see what will come of it, it is this child' " (p. 102). When Dr. Ferris expresses skepticism about Nan's interest in medicine, the girl's guardian explains that she has an unconscious talent for medical matters that he intends to nurture without undue force: " 'I don't care whether it's a man's work or a woman's work; if it is hers I'm going to help her the very best way I can. I don't talk to her of course; she's much too young; but I watch her and mean to put the things in her way that she seems to reach out for and try to find' " (pp. 106–7).

Because Dr. Leslie is able to give his ward the chance to strengthen her interest in medicine without discouraging her by imposing society's artificial limitations upon her aspirations, the young girl is able to grow to adolesence strong in her commitment to be a doctor. That commitment wavers during a period of adolescent uncertainty, but it is reaffirmed with added vigor in a scene that is both a turning point in the girl's life and an example of the kind of dedication crucial to the character of the doctor-to-be, regardless of gender.

At loose ends during "the summer which follows the close of her school-life" (p. 158), Nan Prince is torn between her youthful commitment to medicine and her growing realization of how deviant such a commitment is for a young woman to hold. Though she had long been a youthful assistant to her guardian, her apparent interest in such helping wanes as she tries "to fancy herself in sympathy with the conventional world of school and of the everyday ideas of society. And yet her inward sympathy with a doctor's and a surgeon's work grew stronger, though she dismissed reluctantly the possibility of following her bent in any formal way, since, after all, her world seemed to forbid it" (p. 161). Attempting to follow what seem to be the world's dictates, the young woman tries to believe that she can be happy with a conventional life, but she soon realizes that such a life cannot satisfy her.

Suffering a discontent that at the time knew no name, Nan Prince hurries to the farm where her grandmother had reared her and to the riverbank where she had played as a child. Unknowingly she comes to the very spot where her own mother had contemplated suicide years before.

> the miserable suffering woman, who had wearily come to this place to end their lives, had turned away that the child might make her own choice between the good and evil things of life. Though Nan told herself that she must make it plain how she could spend her time in Oldfields to good purpose and be of most use at home, and must get a new strength for these duties, a decision suddenly presented itself to her with a force of reason and necessity the old dream of it never had shown. Why should it not be a reality that she studied medicine? (pp. 165–66)

What had been a childhood dream, nurtured by the careful upbringing of Dr. Leslie, takes on the added dimension of adult choice and dedication. The crucial element here is that of medicine as Nan's *calling*, the very element that crystallizes her decision and that will give her sufficient intensity of purpose to carry it out. Jewett describes the turning point in the girl's life in a way that demonstrates yet another strain in the makeup of the ideal doctor, the strain of a religious-like calling to the work at hand, in short, the God-given will to be a doctor:

> The thought entirely possessed her . . . Her whole heart went out to this work, and she wondered why she had ever lost sight of it. She was sure this was the way in which she could find most happiness. God had directed her at last, and though the opening of her sealed orders had been long delayed, the suspense had only made her surer that she must hold fast this unspeakably great motive: something to work for with all her might as long as she lived. People might laugh or object. Nothing should turn her aside, and a new affection for kind and patient Dr. Leslie filled her mind . . . her former existence seemed like a fog and uncertainty of death, from which she had turned away, this time of her own accord, toward a great light of satisfaction and certain safety and helpfulness. (pp. 166–67)

This new-found will and God-given direction help Nan to strengthen her determination and provide the foundation for her apprenticeship to Dr. Leslie. Her zeal and pride also wear down the resistance of those around her who had first jeered; they come at last to accept her studies and ambition "as inevitable and a matter of course, even if they do not actively approve" (p. 183).

Dr. Leslie teaches Nan all that he can. Aware of her own ignorance, Nan soon learns "that it is resource, and bravery, and being able to think for one's self, that make a physician worth anything." She realizes that "there is something needed beside even drill and experience; every student of medicine should be fitted by nature with a power of insight, a gift for his business, for knowing what is the right thing to do and the right time to do it; must have this God-given power in his own nature of using and discovering the resources of medicine without constant reliance upon the books or the fashion" (pp. 184–85).

In Nan Prince's apprenticeship, Jewett shows the ideal course of a doctor's preparation and demonstrates the importance of the right kind of character to the successful completion of that training. After nearly two years of tutelage with the old country doctor, however, both Nan Prince and Dr. Leslie realize that it is time for her to enter medical school. In delineating the young woman's medical school experience, Jewett shows the difficulties faced not only by Nan Prince but also by any woman who would commit herself to a professional career at a time when the varied support systems available to men were systematically denied to women. Jewett's presentation of the difficulties facing Nan is cogent and characterizes her further by showing her overcoming substantial obstacles, among them some of the more questionable characteristics of the male medical establishment:

If a young man plans the same course, everything conspires to help him and forward him, and the very fact of his having chosen one of the learned professions gives him a certain social preeminence and dignity. But in the days of Nan's student life, it was just the reverse. Though she had been directed toward such a purpose entirely by her single talent, instead of by the motives of expediency which rule the decisions of a large proportion of the young men who study medicine, she found little encouragement either from the quality of the school or the interest of society in general. (pp. 192–193)

Yet, as apprehensive as she is, Nan's dedication and intensity of purpose overcome her qualms:

when she remembered her perfect certainty that she was doing the right thing ... there was no real drawing back, but rather a proud certainty of her most womanly and respectable calling, and a reverent desire to make the best possible use of the gifts God had certainly not made a mistake in giving her. "If He meant I should be a doctor," the girl told herself, "the best thing I can do is to try to be a good one." (p. 193)

Once Nan Prince is in medical school, Jewett shifts the novel's focus to introduce Miss Anna Prince, Nan's aunt, in her moneyed and leisurely life in Dunport, a life that is held out, along with the possibility of marriage, as the last temptation and final obstacle that Nan must reject and surmount before her dedication to her medical career is fully formed and invincible. Miss Prince has long been estranged from the girl, but upon receiving a brief note from Nan asking if she might take one of her vacations from medical school and visit Dunport, the lonely old lady relents. She and her niece are reconciled and the two soon become fast friends. Nan's stay in Dunport is pleasant, and she enjoys the wealth and leisure and the attentions of the young lawyer, George Gerry, whom her aunt hopes she will marry. She does not, however, enjoy the disapproval generated by her announcement that she does indeed intend to be a doctor, and she is annoyed that the disapproval of her aunt and the dismay of George Gerry carry with them the assumption that her decision is a short-lived caprice. She feels that "it would have been better to have been violently opposed than to have been treated like a child whose foolish whim would soon be forgotten when anything better offered itself" (p. 255).

In spite of her annoyance at being taken for granted in her most vital decision, Nan grows fonder and fonder of her aunt and of George Gerry, so fond in fact that she extends her visit long beyond the time originally planned. By this means, Jewett is able to give added depth to Nan Prince's character by showing what she will have to give up for her career. At a tea party given by Mrs. Fraley, a friend of Nan's aunt, Nan is told by her hostess in no uncertain terms that a woman's place is in the home and that a strong-minded woman is out of place and unwelcome everywhere. Nan's rejoinder begins with an objection to the " 'habit of using strong-mindedness as a term of rebuke' " (p. 279). She goes on in considerable detail to speak of her belief in herself and her frustration at being forced to apologize for studying medicine.

"I believe that God has given me a fitness for it [,she says.]... Nobody persuaded me into following such a plan; I simply grew toward it. And I have everything to learn, and a great many faults to overcome, but I am trying to get on as fast as may be... But everything helps the young man to follow his bent; he has an honored place in society, and because he is a student of one of the learned professions, he ranks above the men who follow other pursuits. I don't see why it should be a shame and dishonor to a girl who is trying to do the same thing and to be of equal use to the world. God would not give us the same talents if what were right for men were wrong for women." (pp. 281–82)

Though able to defend herself with relative ease against the constricted expectations of the larger society, Nan is less able to ward off the onslaught of love that she fears will finally undermine her dedication to medicine. After a particularly enjoyable evening with her suitor, the young woman endures a sleepless night of self-doubt during which her resolve is again tested, this time more severely than ever before. Though weakened by Jewett's inability to render it dramatically, the scene is nonetheless a telling presentation of Nan Prince's strength and her ability to prevail over the most intensely personal obstacle she has yet encountered. She envisions a domestic life and feels that her dream of a medical career no longer matters as her old ambitions fall away and are replaced by thoughts of marriage and homemaking:

But as the night waned, the certainty of her duty grew clearer and clearer... she must not marry... her duty was not this, and a certainty that satisfaction and the blessing of God would not follow her into these reverenced and honored limits came to her distinctly... She had not thought she should be able to resist this temptation, but since it had come she was glad she was strong enough to meet it. It would be no real love for another person, and no justice to herself, to give up her work, even though holding it fast would bring weariness and pain and reproach, and the loss of many things that other women hold dearest and best. (pp. 307–8)

Having passed through her dark night of uncertainty, Nan Prince is able to refuse George Gerry's offer of marriage, even though she is very fond of him. Again, her refusal is cast in religious terms as she speaks to the downcast young man about her sense of mission saying, "I don't know why God should have made me a doctor, so many other things have seemed fitter for a woman; but I see the blessedness of such a useful life more and more every year, and I am very thankful for such a trust. It is a splendid thing to have the use of any gift of God. It isn't for us to choose again, or wonder and dispute, but just work in our own places, and leave the rest to God' " (p. 327).

Soon after withstanding this final temptation, Nan returns to Oldfields and decides to decline appointments to several city hospitals and not to study abroad but rather to remain and continue to study with Dr. Leslie whom she knows is the best teacher she can find. In explaining her refusal of marriage, the young woman talks candidly to her mentor, saying, " 'Now that I look back at it all I am so glad to have had those days; I shall work better all my life for having been able to make myself perfectly sure that I know my way' " (pp. 339–40). Greatly pleased by her declaration, the old country doctor thinks warmly of the young woman who had been his ward, his pupil, his close friend, and who would in time be his colleague. In his musings, he compares her choice of calling to Christ's, thinking, "she had come to her work as Christ came to his, not to be ministered unto but to minister" (p. 340).

Thus, Nan Prince becomes both doctor and minister, and in so doing becomes even more highly idealized. In the final scene, the young country doctor visits the familiar and beloved riverbank. In the quiet interlude, it is clear that the young woman who has succeeded so well in her resolve to become a doctor will succeed equally well now that she had begun her professional life:

> presently she went closer to the river, and looked far across it and beyond it to the hills. The eagles swung to and fro above the water, but she looked beyond them into the sky. The soft air and the sunshine came close to her; the trees stood about and seemed to watch her; and suddenly she reached her hands upward in an ecstasy of life and strength and gladness. "O God," she said, "I thank thee for my future." (pp. 350–51)

In Nan Prince, Jewett takes the ideal character of the doctor several steps beyond what Holmes, Mitchell, and Howells had established. To the catalog of virtues already evident in earlier fictional doctors, Jewett adds the singular elements of God-given calling, will, and dedication. The very best doctor is born to medicine, is (whether woman or man) a chosen individual whose true calling is to be a healer. In that calling, which transcends issues of gender, she or he ministers to both body and spirit, and in so ministering goes beyond being just a good doctor to become the even more ideal doctor-priest. Thus, with Dr. Leslie and Nan Prince, the two exemplars of the country doctor, readers found a fully established and powerful idealization to remember and to look back to in their everyday dealings with their own doctors.

What that image would become in the next half-century and more is firmly anchored in the portrayals of Jewett and her predecessors. What they established became the basis for an evolving American type, a fictionalized dream character that in the coming decades of the twentieth century would take on various overtones and shadings while remaining essentially an ideal writ large. Though removed further and further from the reality of everyday life, that ideal and its evocative power would maintain an extraordinarily tenacious hold on the imaginations and hopes of the American public—patients and their doctors alike.

6

Literary Artifacts: Continuations

THE TENACIOUS IMAGE

Among American writers and their readers, the popularity of the idealized doctor as a fictional type continued during the closing decades of the nineteenth century and grew even greater throughout the twentieth century. The medical novels of Holmes, Mitchell, Howells, and Jewett established the germinal image of the benevolent doctor of good character. Other writers—from the worst to the best—would take up that image, examine it, and embellish its familiar contours, decade by decade, until they had produced a collective idealization that would live on in spite of its excesses and inaccuracies.

The continuation of the literary and cultural tradition established in the medical novels of the American Romantics and Realists was aided by the fact that writers of all sorts incorporated the idealized doctor into their fictional worlds. Thus readers of all sorts were exposed to an increasingly diverse range of variations on a crucial icon. At one end of the spectrum, the doctor as central character has appeared in some of the most easily forgotten of American novels. Yet regardless of how flawed the novel, in most cases the doctor at its center is portrayed as an essentially flawless individual, dedicated to healing both the physical and emotional ills of patients and often providing advice about the solutions to nonmedical problems. Characteristic of these problem-solving doctors is the title character of George Washington Cable's 1883 novel, *Dr. Sevier*, written between the years when Howells created Dr. Breen and Jewett presented Dr. Leslie and Nan Prince. Cable's work, set in New Orleans, is cumbersomely plotted, melodramatic, and overburdened with his unsuccessful attempt to approx-imate a southern dialect for his characters.

Of these characters, it is John Richling (the prodigal son of a Kentucky gentleman) and his northern wife, Mary, who are at the novel's center and the recipients of the medical skill, compassion, and generosity of Dr. Sevier, who is most fully characterized in his relationship with them. Having saved the life of Mary Richling, who reminds him of his dead wife Alice, Sevier (early described as a doctor who "laid his left hand on the rich and his right hand on the poor; and who was not left-handed")[1] finds his solitary life increasingly entwined with the Richling's activities and declining fortunes. At first he is annoyed, then interested, and finally he befriends them and becomes their confidant and ally.

As the relationship between the good doctor and the Richlings grows, Sevier becomes a warmer and more humane person. Earlier in the novel, Cable characterizes the doctor as an austere, pure-minded man who is "fixedly untender everywhere, except—but always except—in the sick cham-ber." Although his inner heart is "all of flesh," Sevier's demands for the "rectitude of mankind" make him harsh and impatient with the follies of others. Just as he opposes folly and evil, so does he—in expectable fashion—wage "war against malady. To fight; to stifle; to cut down; to uproot; to overwhelm,—these were his springs of action" (pp. 6–7).

The novel chronicles the growth of Sevier, not as a doctor per se but as a humanitarian. Cable seems willing to take Sevier's doctoring for granted, referring to it infrequently and then only briefly. Of more concern is the mellowing of Sevier's austere, lonely, and frowning character, a mellowing that is evident as he learns from the Richlings that kindness and compassion can go hand-in-hand with his dedicated battle against sickness and evil. It is the Richlings who come to understand Sevier's "frowning good intention" (p. 293), and in their need they provide the doctor with the chance to escape from his loneliness by helping them. Having lent Richling money, helped him to find work, and arranged to have him released from prison, Sevier comes to learn, as he tells his friend, that " 'the poor are a godsend to the rich. They're set over against each other to keep pity and mercy and charity in the human heart' " (p. 447). Once Sevier's already admirable character is further enhanced by this learned lesson, Cable can allow Richling to die and the novel to come rapidly to a close. In the midst of a melodramatic and cumbersome fictional world, Sevier becomes, via his humanization, a more admirable character than when his devotion to healing was coupled with a harsh and less altruistic temperament.

Even more melodramatic and contrived is Mary E. Wilkins-Freeman's *Doc Gordon*, published in 1906. Here the title character, predictably wise and benevolent, plays the role of experienced teacher to the neophyte doctor, James Elliot.[2] The good doctor is also counselor to the younger Elliot about his courtship of Clemency Ewing, whose ostensible identity as Gordon's niece is revealed as part of a well-intentioned scheme to protect the girl from learning of her own sordid background. Out of that background and into the life of the girl and her protector, the good doctor, comes her deranged father, a man who is "a very devil incarnate" (p. 105). As the melodrama mounts, Doc Gordon inadvertently kills the girl's menacing father but is exonerated in the reader's eyes because of circumstances and because he meant no harm. Wilkins-Freeman, herself a doctor's wife, surrounds her protagonist with an unconvincing air of mystery arising from questions about his own wife's supposed death and the contrived revelation that Mrs. Ewing, supposedly Clemency's mother and Gordon's widowed sister, is in fact his wife who has kept her true identity a secret to all those who had thought her dead (pp. 224–25). In a thoroughly unconvincing conclusion, Doc Gordon gives his wife, who is in great pain from a terminal disease, a fatal overdose of morphine (p. 260). The moral questions raised here are readily answered in a concocted happy ending that reasserts the doctor's innate goodness and returns him to the community's good graces. Memorable for little else, *Doc Gordon* does demonstrate that even in the hands of the poorest of writers, the figure of the benevolent and fundamentally good doctor remains a recognizable type, even when it is portrayed in the most hackneyed and unrealistic manner.

Equal to *Doc Gordon* in its degree of contrivance is *Doctor Nye of North Ostable*, [3] written by Joseph C. Lincoln and published in 1923. The novel recounts the rising fortunes of Ephraim Nye, another doctor of good character, who has been severely wronged by his fellow-townspeople. Lincoln establishes an initial air of mystery that soon turns to unabashed melodrama as the "scandalous story" of the "queer critter," Nye, is hinted at and then explained (p. 27). The doctor had years before been accused of embezzling funds from the Congregationalist Church building fund, of which he was treasurer. An initial denial followed by an unexplained admission of guilt thoroughly confuse the people of North Ostable because Nye "was—well, he was kind of a—a President of the United States in this town and they couldn't, the most of them, believe he was a thief" (p. 36).

Lincoln's plot thickens as Nye's wife, Fanny, well known for her extravagance, dies in the midst of the furor about the theft. Her older brother (just coincidentally the town's respected judge) blames Nye for her death and vengefully forces his arrest for theft. Nye is convicted and, thus, in the novel's present-time, he is the prodigal returning after more than five years. The process by which he comes to reclaim his rightful place comprises the central action of the book, and in his machinations to restore his reputation he is revealed as a thoroughly good man and dedicated healer who has been greviously wronged.

Nye's character is embellished with numerous melodramatic trappings. He has "a kind of devilish fascination about him that attracted everyone, especially the women" (p. 42), and in keeping with that fascination, he had, between his release from prison and his return to North Ostable, served as a surgeon in the French Army. Balancing these exotic elements in his resolve to return in order to clear himself in the eyes of others (p. 62).

Nye's determination sets into motion a series of events that keep the novel boiling along. He refuses a bribe from Judge Copeland to leave town (p. 67), treats the first of his new patients for free, and once word has spread he gets more patients who seldom pay in full. "And, pay or no pay, he was thoroughly enjoying these opportunities to practice always his beloved profession" (p. 84). Here in his love for medicine, Nye is reminiscent of Nan Prince with her dedication to healing. In Nye's case, that dedication and his skill soon meet their test as he successfully treats his landlord's wife for typhoid and vows to track down the source of the disease.

In his quest, Nye, at first only intent upon clearing his own name, follows his altruistic instincts and works to alleviate the problems of others. Among them is his niece, Judge Copeland's daughter Faith, whose life Nye saves and whose romance with young Tom Stone he eventually aids, over the judge's objections. In his willingness to stand up against Judge Copeland, Nye, the dedicated healer, is portrayed as self-reliant, honest, and highly individualistic. He is the complete doctor.

Adding coincidence to contrivance, Lincoln, in an apparent attempt to present all of Nye's best qualities, introduces a romantic subplot via Katherine Powell, the doctor's first and true love, who also conveniently returns to North Ostable, pursues him quietly, and calculatedly becomes his advocate before the skeptical townspeople (pp. 218–19). Freighted as it is with melodramatic trappings and subplots and in need of an external force to tie up its loose ends, and the novel receives from Lincoln a finale growing out of a typhoid epidemic, which strikes rich and poor alike and allows Dr. Nye, through his unstinting labors, to re-establish his good name.

Because of his dedicated and expert service, the once-disgraced doctor becomes known as "the miracle man" (p. 333). Furthermore, he clears his good name (he had shielded his wife who had stolen the church's money), convinces Judge Copeland to stop interfering in Faith's romance, and in the closing scenes is reunited with Katherine Powell. In short, love, honesty, dedication, and the healer's true spirit triumph, and Ephraim Nye is restored to his rightful place of honor in an admiring town.

Equally honorable, though mired in an even more inferior fictional world, is Dr. Richard Oakland, hero of George J. Zaffiras' *The Doctor From Iowa* (1949). At times virtually unreadable, the novel paints as glowing and stereotyped a picture of the young, idealistic country doctor as can be found. Affluent and altruistic, Oakland is devoted to his ailing and domineering mother (" 'I don't need a wife . . . [he says], I have my mother.' ")[4] and dedicated to serving his patients in Cornville, Iowa, "well, honorably, and faithfully" (p. 16).

As he ministers to his patients, the young doctor becomes involved with a young Indian woman who is trying to help organize the local coal miners. Dismayed by his own interest in her, Oakland reminds himself futilely that "a doctor must keep his dignity" (p. 170), but his resolve to avoid the young woman melts as she stirs his sense of justice by her work on the miners' behalf. Asserting his individuality and growing even more admirable in his new-found autonomy, Dr. Oakland decides to help the miners, falls in love, and manages to maintain his professional image throughout the novel.

In the service of a happy ending, he is saved from what he believes may be a marriage damaging to his career by the discovery that the troublesome Indian woman is neither an Indian nor trouble. Rather, she reveals herself to be the rightful owner of the coal mines, which she will, with Oakland's help, set to working properly. Able to assert his own altruistic and individualistic nature, the good young doctor gains a wife and a social conscience, both of which augment his admirable and idealized character.

For all its flaws and excesses, the novel invokes and capitalizes upon already familiar patterns. Oakland's competence is presented as a given, and he becomes more admirable, not because he becomes a more expert doctor but because he becomes a more concerned and committed person. Again, the doctor of good character becomes all the more laudable as he extends the impulse to help others from a constricted medical sphere to the more broadly based social world of which he is a part.

The importance of the doctor's social concerns and altruistic involvement with larger elements of society extending beyond the world of patients is also evident in the medical fiction of some of America's better writers. Among these novelists, the idealized doctor is a commonplace character, similar to the type already established in American fiction. In some of these better novels, there is less focus on the doctor as medical practitioner than on the doctor as the embodiment of particular thematic concerns; in other of the better novels, the doctor as doctor, already a familiar type, appears in the forefront again and again.

In Robert Herrick's turn-of-the-century novel, *The Web of Life* (1900), there is a blend of the doctor as practitioner and doctor as thematic embodiment. The young and idealistic surgeon, Dr. Sommers, "the ornament of the Surgical Ward at St. Isidore's"[5] is the central character of the novel that chronicles the effects of his decision not to pursue a wealthy clientele but rather to practice medicine among the poor and needy. Although banal in its plotting, the story is enlivened and intensified by Herrick's lean and taut prose, which is able to evoke mood and a sense of person and place with vivid economy.

Sommers's individualistic decision to strike out on his own and to foreswear the help of the wealthy Hitchcocks, who want to "bring him a little closer to [the influential members] of his profession" (p. 25), leads him to a life of grinding and brutalizing poverty. His dedication to help those in need is sorely tested by patients who have little understanding or appreciation of what he does for them. Deeply in love with and married to the widow of a man whose life he had saved earlier, Sommers is unable to find in love and marriage an adequate shield against his growing disenchantment with his chosen life. He is happy with his wife, but the isolated happiness of love is not enough.

What Sommers learns is the need for balance, for satisfaction and a reasonable reward for the work he does and loves. He is unable to be the kind of competent and dedicated doctor he desires in the midst of overly adverse conditions, and so, after the suicide of his beloved wife, he strikes out in a new direction. Sommers "resolved to find service in one of the military hospitals that before long became notorious as pestholes. From the day he arrived in Tampa, he found enough to tax all his energies in trying to save the lives of raw troops" (p. 331).

In such service the talented and dedicated doctor rediscovers his own sense of purpose as well as a new maturity that enables him to resolve the ethical questions that plagued him regarding the relationship between wealth and influence and genuine service and altruism. He comes to recognize that wealth and the power it allows can be beneficial if they are dedicated to the care of others. Having resolved these issues, he is now free to marry the wealthy Louise Hitchcock, who supports him in his decision to work with the general practitioner, Dr. Knowles, in an "old-fashioned and common-place practice" (p. 349). Further exemplifying his newly matured altruism is his ability to see that Hitchcock money need not be summarily rejected, but, rather, can be put to good use: "It did not take Louise and Sommers long...to convince Colonel Hitchcock that they were absolutely sincere in the decision [not to accept Louise's inheritance] and to interest him in methods of returning his wealth, at his death, to the world" (p. 353). By the novel's conclusion, weakened by its reliance on a banal happy ending, Herrick has brought his idealistic young doctor full circle. Having once rejected the wealth of Louise Hitchcock, Sommers comes to accept that wealth for its potential to do good on a large scale, just as he, the compassionate doctor, does a similar good on a more limited, personal scale.[6]

This tension between individual service and self-satisfaction and altruism is also crucial in John Steinbeck's *In Dubious Battle* (1936), the record of a strike among apple pickers in California's Torgas Valley in the early 1930's. Here, the good and able Doc Burton is a background figure representing a man who is concerned about injustice but unable to commit himself to either the status quo of the growers or the new order of the strikers to whom he ministers.

Steinbeck uses the doctor as a choric figure, a commentator on the action, and shows that Doc Burton's desire for scientific detachment and objectivity, for clear vision unencumbered by emotional involvement or personal concern is an untenable stance. Unlike Holmes's doctors who put their clear sight to immediate use in the service of their patients, Doc Burton wants "to be able to look at the whole thing" without what he feels are the "blinders of agreement."[7] For Steinbeck, though, people must eventually commit themselves (as did Herrick's Dr. Sommers). To refuse to do so is to refuse to be fully human, and Doc Burton, good doctor though he is, finally disappears from the novel one night as he goes off from the strikers' camp to visit a patient. In his use and final disposition of Burton, Steinbeck makes clear that there is no place in the world for the indecisive and un-committed individual, regardless of his or her other virtues.

The self-destruction caused by isolation and the inability to commit one-self to an ideal is also treated in the evocative novel, *The Heart Is A Lonely Hunter* (1940) by Carson McCullers.[8] Unusual in its presentation of a black doctor, the book centers on the quest for meaning and fulfillment of several characters who try to learn from the central character, a young mute who serves as a catalyst in their lives. One of the searchers is Benedict Copeland, the dedicated and skilled doctor who is, at last, unable to hunt out the meaning of things and equally unable to cope with the world in which he lives.

Copeland's isolation, similar to Doc Burton's, leads him to a metaphoric rather than an actual disappearance. Unable to resolve the questions that gnaw at him, even as he works to heal others, Copeland is unable to heal himself by quieting the loneliness in his own heart. Though different from the medical fiction focusing on the idealized doctor, this novel, as did Stein-beck's, demonstrates the varied use to which the good doctor of admirable traits has been put in American fiction.

More traditional in its use of the doctor than either the novel of McCullers or Steinbeck is John O'Hara's novelette, *A Family Party* (1956), "a sten-ographic report of an address by Mr. Albert W. Shoemaker . . . at a dinner in honor of Dr. Samuel G. Merritt"[9] upon his retirement after forty years of practice in Lyons, Pennsylvania. By using the device of a spoken testi-monial, O'Hara achieves considerable emphasis via the compression of Dr. Merritt's lifetime into its laudatory retelling. More importantly, by having the testimonial delivered by one of the doctor's many patients, O'Hara is able to present a patient's view of the popular doctor's achievements.

Those achievements, expectably familiar, form a catalog of virtues that establish Merritt as a worthy successor to the idealized general practitioners of Holmes and Jewett. Known by everyone in town, Sam Merritt is always the first one to arrive when needed (p. 11), and his unstinting service is matched by his lack of concern with money and payment for his work (p. 25). His philanthropic nature is an outgrowth of his altruistic decision to become a doctor, a decision that had been precipitated by the death of his brother (p. 34).

In the speaker's description, Dr. Merritt exhibits the best characteristics of the family doctor: " 'The majority of us here tonight have felt the touch of his hand on our pulse or had him tell us to say "Ah" and do all the things a family doctor does in the course of his daily routine' " (p. 41). Yet even more to his credit, Merritt goes far beyond the routine. He is " 'more than a doctor' "; he is " 'a man that the thing he wanted most in the world was for [people] to get well' " (p. 42).

Not only does Merritt minister to his patients with sufficient intensity of purpose grounded in selflessness, but he also manifests a degree of social concern that links him to the doctors created by Cable, Lincoln, Zaffiras, Herrick, and others. Knowing full well that his town is greatly in need of a hospital, Merritt begins a one-man campaign to raise funds. Out of his own savings and with a loan on his house and a donation from his mother and his sisters, he puts together $ 25,000 and then raises another $ 175,000 through his relentless efforts. In a particularly effective piece of characterization, O'Hara points up Merritt's altruism and social concern by having him accept a necessary compromise and turn over the $200,000 he has raised to a group that goes on to build the needed hospital, not in Lyons but in nearby Johnsville, eight miles away (p. 54).

As if all of this is not enough to establish Merritt as the warmly remembered ideal, O'Hara adds the element of privately borne grief to the catalog of the doctor's virtues. Thinking that the family party is an appropriate place to reveal a family secret, the speaker, Shoemaker, tells of the little-known mental breakdown of the doctor's beloved wife, Alice, and of Merritt's quiet suffering and devoted care of her. To conclude his testimonial and to demonstrate the love and high regard that the townspeople feel for their ideal doctor, Shoemaker presents Sam Merritt with the $20,000 gift that the town has raised for the maternity ward at Johnsville Hospital " 'to be known as the Alice C. Merritt Ward' " (p. 64). Thus personal grief merges with public good, and O'Hara provides a means of rebirth and immortality for his carefully drawn ideal.

Equally ideal but a doctor of a far different sort is Samuel Abelman, the title character of Gerald Green's *The Last Angry Man* (1956). Around for more than forty years, Abelman (aptly though obviously named) is "too old and tired for night work,"[10] but that fact does not keep his nonpaying patients from rousting him out of bed to care for a girl who has been beaten and dumped on his front stoop. For his patients, Abelman the G.P. must always be available: " 'Dr. Baumgart is an *internist* [one yells] . . . He don't make no night calls. You just a doctor for everyday kind of work' " (p. 6).

Nearing the end of almost half-a-century of such "everyday kind of work," Abelman will also have his testimonial, but it will be no family party like that given for Sam Merritt. Instead, the healer of the poor and the dispossessed of his decaying Brooklyn neighborhood will be honored by a television special designed in the hope of saving a large advertising account. In this unlikely mating of media hype and idealized doctoring, Green establishes a tension that serves to illuminate both Abelman's world and that of Woodrow ("Woody") Thrasher, the television executive whose desperation about possibly losing a lucrative account gives rise to the idea of honoring the aging doctor in the first show of an "Americans, U.S.A." series. Fighting for his own professional survival, Thrasher sets out to use Abelman and comes to admire and finally to love the angry old man. What Thrasher learns as he prepares the show provides Green with an effective device for presenting Abelman both in the present time of the novel and in retrospect, and the portrait that emerges is as much an idealization as any of those painted in the preceding decades.

Fortunately for Thrasher's media-oriented sensibility, Abelman looks the part of the ideal G.P. with a "strong, hard face... forehead [that] was high ...lips firm and thin" (pp. 35–36). Conveniently for the TV man, Abelman has, in his small backyard garden, a tree that is a metaphor for his own life, a Lombardy poplar "of regal proportions... that had thrived amidst so much filth and squalor" (p. 30). Abelman himself, though, is beyond thriving. He has lost his poor patients to dispensaries and free clinics and he has seen his richer patients desert him in favor of more expensive specialists (p. 47). In spite of such losses, he goes on, totally engrossed in his work. "He loved the ritual of the office; opening the double-doors to the examining room, inviting the next patient in; the case histories, the preliminary interrogations, the probings" (p. 151). Not only does he love the forms and the rituals of healing, but Abelman also loves his patients, a fact scoffed at by his friend and colleague Max Vogel, who is one of Thrasher's informants and a spokesman for the traditionally closed fraternal world of medicine: "Vogel jerked a thumb in the direction of his friend and spoke to Thrasher and Daws. 'It's not that he's so honest, fellahs, he's just stupid. He makes friends out of patients, the worst thing you can do. Patients should be scared stiff of their doctors' " (p. 188).

Thrasher also learns of Abelman's initial decision to study medicine, a decision rejoiced in by his father who for years contributed fifty cents a day to his son's medical school expenses (p. 187) and who died while Abelman was studying for and taking an exam (p. 207). Shocked by his own disregard of his dying father, Abelman, who after two-and-a-half years of medical school "had not lost his feeling of arrival, of initiation into some blessed fraternity," (p. 200) decides to give up medicine. His decision, growing out of grief and a desire for atonement, is countered by his fiancee, Sarah, who tells him pointedly that if he doesn't continue at Bellevue he can stop seeing her (p. 211).

From Abelman's own reminiscences, Thrasher learns of the influence of Harlow Brooks, a Bellevue professor who had also encouraged Abelman to continue his studies. It was Brooks who had described the art of healing in the very terms that Abelman would actualize in his own work (and in terms that echo the words of Green's predecessors in the making of a collective myth): " 'Medicine [Brooks had said] isn't drugs and surgery and therapy. Medicine is people. We deal with people, each one different, valuable, worthy of some kind of special attention.' " (p. 216).

In his involvement with people, Abelman is most fully idealized. Thrasher learns from Sarah Abelman about her continual wondering " 'if other doctors reacted so personally to illness. Each new case Sam took on became part of him, for better or for worse, eating a little bit of him away, eroding his character and his strong body' " (p. 254). Yet for all of his involvement with and for all he does for his patients, Abelman is rewarded not with their loyalty but all too often with their capriciousness. As he grows older, he loses those patients who want a young, more modern doctor, one like Seymour Baumgart who is "neat, cool, and aloof in a white coat, a model of professional competence who charged them twice as much, made no effort to become friends with them, and looked over their heads when he spoke" (p. 423).

For Woody Thrasher, himself humanized by his contact with Sam Abelman, the electronic biography at first conceived of as a gimmick becomes a far more significant thing. "All [Thrasher] could offer was a television program, but maybe it would be the best revenge of all—someone had to prove to the Baumgarts of the world that the Sam Abelmans were also rewarded" (p. 425). The reward, though, is not to be seen by the ideal doctor who has earned it. Abelman dies of a massive heart attack only hours before the testimonial to him is to be aired.

Once the last angry man is dead, the novel loses much of its power. Green allows Abelman's death to become, via television's exploitation, a triumph for the medium and a bittersweet success for Woody Thrasher, who, against his better instincts, is led to intone platitudes about the "multiform" uses of "the word" that could "debauch and deceive" but could also "be used to create and uplift" (p. 494). The tawdry media denouement fails, however, to diminish the real power of the story of Dr. Sam Abelman. Though different in externals from the ideal doctors of Holmes, Jewett, Herrick, or O'Hara, Abelman is a worthy recipient of the mantle of dedicated competence and altruism that had been passed down from one generation of fictional doctors to another.

That mantle is also worn by the doctors created by some of America's best novelists (although their idealized healers do not always appear in the best of their fiction). The physicians created by James, Anderson, Faulkner, and Fitzgerald do not function in quite the same straightforward manner as do their counterparts in lesser American novels. Whereas the ideal figure created by these best novelists has much in common with other fictional doctors, it is generally used for different purposes. Rather than just celebrate the doctor's best traits and most laudable actions, these writers place their fictional healers in complex social worlds in which they become integral parts in an overall fictional design. This use of the doctor for particular thematic purposes is notably true of Henry James's *The Wings of the Dove*, published in 1902. Usually ranked among the best of his work, the novel is a striking exercise in the manipulation of point of view. James's heroine is a young American heiress, Milly Theale, who goes to Europe in order to experience the world more fully, to take "full in the face the whole assault of life."[11] Ironically, as she pursues life, she carries with her the germ of an idea that she is dying, and inevitably for James's purposes, the very idea, carried to obsessional lengths, kills her.

Essential to the working out of the young woman's fatal delusion and to the success of James's fictional design are the various people whom Milly Theale meets and is affected by; through them, the reader comes to know her just as she, accepting too readily others' views of her, comes distortedly to know herself. In his Preface to the New York Edition of the novel, James writes explicitly of his plan for "the *indirect* presentation of his main image," saying that he will watch her "as it were, through the successive windows of other people's interest in her" (p. xxii).

Among the "successive windows that provide a multifaceted view of Milly Theale, the most direct (the straightest) view is provided by Sir Luke Strett, the English doctor who treats her mysterious illness. Strett, "the greatest of medical lights," (p. 168) is a "great beneficent being" (p. 382) who, as a skilled and sympathetic observer of patients, is the reader's major source of accurate information about Milly Theale. At their first visit Milly knows that he will find out "simply by his genius...literally everything" about her (p. 175), and he does just that. Realizing that she is quite well, except for her morbid fancy, he advises her to accept life and happiness, telling her, " 'Worry about nothing. You *have* at least no worries' " (pp. 180–182). Such advice, though, is the very thing that Milly cannot follow, even when Strett tells her that " 'to live [is] exactly what I'm trying to persuade you to take the trouble to do' " (p. 183).

In spite of Strett's perceptive advice, Milly's lack of self-knowledge, coupled with her obsession that she is indeed a "dove" as her confidante Kate Croy calls her (p. 210), lead to her self-destruction. For all his beneficent skill, Strett is helpless before Milly Theale's belief in her own imminent death, just as Dr. Kittredge was helpless before Elsie Venner's antenatal inheritance. Yet Strett's inability to help Milly break out of her delusion is no reflection on his own competence. Rather, it is a crucial means by which James emphasizes the powerful hold that the young woman's delusion exerts on her. Seen by the reader through the distorted views that others have of her (views based on the self-interested uses to which those others put her), Milly Theale comes to be the *self-less* creation of those who manipulate her to their own ends. Only Sir Luke Strett, studying her in order to help her, can penetrate her dovelike facade and approach the truth about the dying young woman. That truth—that she can live if only she wills to and if she accepts life whole—is also available to the reader, but it is not available to the young woman whose warped view of herself finally leads her to turn "her face to the wall" (p. 427) and die.[12]

The warped sense of self and consequent isolation that lead to Milly Theale's death are also found in Sherwood Anderson's *Winesburg, Ohio* (1919). Although stylistically the polar opposite from James, Anderson also embodies in his work similar thematic concerns that demonstrate the destructive effects of living in the world without adequate self-knowledge. The thematic kinship of the two is apparent in Anderson's dedication of *Winesburg* to his mother who "first awoke in [him] the hunger to see beneath the surface of lives."[13]

In *Winesburg*, Anderson portrays two doctors who provide "successive windows" that allow the reader to see the other inhabitants of Winesburg in a clearer light. Furthermore, by juxtaposing Dr. Reefy and Dr. Parcival, Anderson is able to comment implicitly on the traits that differentiate the two very different healers. Of the two, Dr. Parcival is the antithesis of what a doctor should be; in simplest terms, he is uncaring. Anderson describes him as a man whose "teeth were black and irregular" and about whose eyes "there was something strange" (p. 49). What is strange about Parcival's eyes is that they do not let him see, either himself or the world around him. Unseeing, he is as self-deluded as Milly Theale, and when he befriends George Willard and becomes the young man's self-styled mentor, Parcival can only tell him at great length of the advisability of adopting "a line of conduct that he himself was unable to define" (p. 50).

Parcival can no more define appropriate conduct for young Willard than he can actualize it himself. Like S. Weir Mitchell's inverted images of the ideal doctor, Parcival is the antithesis of what a doctor should be. Having come to medicine after being a reporter and after having studied to be a Presbyterian minister, Parcival had arrived in Winesburg drunk, had announced himself a doctor, and had begun to attract a few, usually nonpaying patients. In his ministering to the poor, though, there is no hint of altruism: quartered in an office that is "unspeakably dirty," Parcival, as he admits to George Willard, does not want patients. What he wants is to write a book that will put into permanent form the tales he tells Willard, tales that "began nowhere and ended nowhere" (pp. 50–51).

Unlike his namesake to whom the Holy Grail was revealed, Dr. Parcival is unable to find meaning within his isolated life, and his interest in George Willard is grounded only in the young man's willingness to listen to the doctor's long-winded tales. The tales exemplify Parcival's self-centered and warped vision, apparent when he advises Willard, saying, " 'I want to fill you with hatred and contempt so that you will be a superior being' " (p. 55).

Ironically, Parcival is as far as possible from being superior, either as a person or as a doctor. Unable to see himself, he cannot help himself, nor can he help others, and Anderson's most negative view of him is reserved for the moment when Parcival refuses to leave his office and attend to a child who has been thrown from a buggy and severely injured. His refusal leads the self-deluded doctor into a paroxysm of fear that the townspeople will come to hang him for his cruel irresponsibility. Shaking with fright, he begs Willard to remember the single idea—the lone truth—that is the basis of Parcival's unwritten book, saying to the youth, " 'The idea is very simple, so simple that if you are not careful you will forget it. It is this—that everyone in the world is Christ and they are all crucified' " (pp. 56–57).

The irony of Parcival's delusion is that rather than the Christ-like figure he imagines himself to be, he is merely another of Winesburg's grotesques who crucifies himself by his self-imposed isolation and removal from the human community. An echo of Hawthorne's isolated healers and as unlike the idealized doctor as is Mitchell's Ezra Wendell, Dr. Parcival is a striking example of the evocative power of the idealized image when it is inverted in order to let its creator achieve particular thematic ends.

Anderson also achieves these thematic ends in his portrayal of Parcival's colleague, the caring and involved Dr. Reefy, who is able to do the very thing—"to see beneath the surface of lives"—that enables him to help others and to live a life far less warped than the lives of the other inhabitants of Winesburg. Although largely forgotten by the town, Reefy can love, and in loving he can break out of his own isolation and minister to others. Although he wears the same suit of clothes for ten years and has only one friend, still in Reefy "there were the seeds of something fine" (pp. 35–36). Those seeds take hold and grow most fully in the intimate relationships that the doctor has, first with his wife and then years later with George Willard's mother. Within these relationships, Reefy the man and Reefy the doctor merge into an insightful and caring person who can minister and bring relief to the barren lives of others.

Reefy's wife, whom he began to court when he was forty-five, had initially come to him as a patient; she was unmarried and pregnant, and after "she came to know Dr. Reefy it seemed to her that she never wanted to leave him again. She went into his office one morning and without her saying anything he seemed to know what had happened to her" (p. 38). The knowledge of the intuitive diagnostician (knowledge of the kind lauded in the fiction of Holmes and Jewett) is joined in Reefy with a good-humored search for truth, a search that is continually begun anew as the searcher, having erected "little pyramids of truth . . . knocked them down again that he might have the truths to erect other pyramids" (p. 35).

Reefy's ability to begin ever anew casts him as the Christ-like figure that Dr. Parcival had only imagined himself to be, and it allows Reefy a perspective on life that keeps him sane in the grotesque world of Winesburg. In his sanity, he is, like Sir Luke Strett, a clear window through which the reader can see without distortion. Just as Reefy provides the reader with a clear point of reference, so does he provide Elizabeth Willard with the chance to see herself and her life more clearly and with less pain. First coming to him as a patient (as years later his wife would first come to him), Elizabeth Willard, unhappily married and tortured by her sense of alienation from those around her, makes of him a confidant and finally a lover.

Together "they talked most of her life, of their two lives and of the ideas that had come to them as they lived their lives in Winesburg." For their several differences, the doctor and his patient are "a good deal alike ... something inside them meant the same thing, wanted the same release, would have left the same impression on the memory of an onlooker" (p. 221). Out of their sameness and their talk comes relief for Elizabeth Willard. "Each time she came to see the doctor ... [she] talked a little more freely and after an hour or two in his presence went down the stairway into Main Street feeling renewed and strengthened against the dullness of her days" (p. 222).

Just as she finds strength and renewal in their talk, Dr. Reefy finds love, and he imagines that as they talk "the woman's body was changing, that she was becoming younger, straighter, stronger" (p. 226). What he imagines of her physical being is a direct analogue of the spiritual renewal that she experiences as a result of the influence of her doctor-lover, a renewal that carries overtones of a religious conversion with Reefy in the role of priest, ministering to his patient-parishioner's spirit. The renewal, though short-lived, strengthens the image of Reefy as a priestly variant of the admirable doctor who brings his clear sight and good character to bear in the service of those in need. In his understanding of and devotion to Elizabeth Willard, Reefy does, in an intensely personal way, the same thing that earlier fictional doctors had done: he reaches out to someone in need, breaks through the debilitating wall of isolation, and ministers to both body and soul.

A similar act of reaching out is central to F. Scott Fitzgerald's *Tender Is The Night*, first published in 1934. In this novel, though, that central action leads to the destruction of the healer rather than to his renewal, because it is not grounded in the clarity of vision that informs Dr. Reefy's care of Elizabeth Willard. Unlike Reefy, the ironically named Dr. Richard Diver fails to dive or to see "beneath the surface of lives," a failing that leads to his own destructive lack of self-knowledge.

What Diver most needs to know is himself, and Fitzgerald takes care to juxtapose his hero's self-centered and increasingly isolated life against what he had once been and might have become. Early in the present time of the novel, Diver, joking with Rosemary Hoyt, the young actress with whom he will eventually have a loveless affair, summarizes his entire life, saying, " 'I'm an old scientist all wrapped up in his private life.' "[14] The statement, both prophetic and truer than Diver realizes, is in direct contrast to what he had been a decade before when he'd been "too valuable, too much of a capital investment" (p. 129) to be sent to war in 1917. Instead, he had gone to Zurich to study to become a psychologist, hoping " 'maybe to be the greatest one that ever lived' " (p. 149).

In Zurich he meets Nicole Warren, the American heiress, whose ostensible schizophrenia and intense fear of men had been triggered by her having been raped by her father. What begins as only a friendship carried on largely by correspondence becomes far more as Diver falls in love with Nicole and reluctantly becomes first her confidant, then her doctor, and finally, in marriage, the center of her life. Aware of the dangers inherent in the relationship, Diver is unable to keep from becoming totally involved: "He tried honestly to divorce her from any obsession that he had stitched her together—glad to see her build up happiness and confidence apart from him; the difficulty was that, eventually, Nicole brought everything to his feet, gifts of sacrificial ambrosia, of worshipping myrtle" (p. 155).

Yet Nicole, whose need is all-consuming, cannot be held responsible for Diver's destruction. He sees all the warnings and knows that he will be consumed, yet he is unable to break away of his own accord. Frequently misread as the story of Nicole's destructive influence on her doctor-husband, the novel actually chronicles Diver's own self-destruction, which is abetted though not caused by his wife's dependence. It is, as Fitzgerald carefully points out, Diver's own dependence and short-sightedness that sow the seeds of his decline. In reaching out to Nicole and in allowing himself to become healer and husband and center of her life for far too long, Diver acts out of his own needs. His fatal weakness and the motive for his charm and for his continually going about "fixing things up" is far from altruistic: "Wanting above all to be brave and kind, he had wanted even more than that to be loved. So it had been" (p. 330).

The excessive self-interest inherent in his root motive of wanting to be loved lets him delude himself that he must always be there to repair Nicole (p. 186) when, in fact, the wiser course would be to let her find her own strength and come to a lessened reliance on him. To do that, though, would weaken, or so Diver believes, the rest of their relationship. Having given so much to her, he is unwilling to risk the loss of Nicole as patient whose illness increasingly defines his professional self, just as her wealth provides and defines the rest of his life. Diver's unwillingness to give up the pathologically interdependent doctor-patient relationship in exchange for one far healthier is based, in part, on his realization that he can never be the great psychologist he had dreamed of being because he is, quite simply, a man of small mind: "Like so many men he had found that he had only one or two ideas—thus his little collection of pamphlets now in its fifteenth German edition contained the germ of all he would ever think or know" (p. 185).

In his realized limitations and even more in his self-interested concern for his most dependent patient, Diver is akin to Mitchell's barren doctor, Ezra Wendell, and as the novel progresses, Diver is increasingly stripped of his ability to do good, either for Nicole or for himself. Unlike Anderson's Dr. Reefy who can renew others and still keep himself intact, Diver lacks the perspective that would allow him to see beneath the surface of his life with

Nicole. He also lacks a social conscience that could allow him to put Nicole's money to good use within a broader social context rather than allow it to become an inescapable trap.

Imprisoned by this inability to see his actions for what they are, Diver acts as the gatekeeper of Nicole's emotional prison from which she strives to escape once she realizes that she is well. Within the shifting balance of their relationship, Nicole, finding herself with new strength, comes to despise having "played planet to Dick's sun" (p. 316) at the very time that he discovers that his own faculties are increasingly weakened (p. 211) and feels "not without desperation...[that] the ethics of his profession [are] dissolving into a lifeless mess" (p. 280).

Not only his ethics, but with increasing rapidity all else about Dick Diver dissolves as Nicole in her growing recovery needs him less and less. No longer the center of her universe, Diver in his every action annoys her more and more (p. 311), and at last as he struggles to save himself, "suddenly, in the space of two minutes, she achieved her victory and justified herself to herself without lie or subterfuge, [and]...cut the cord forever" (p. 329). Faced with Nicole's triumphant independence, Diver realizes that the case is finished and that, finally, he is "at liberty" (p. 329), but his is a liberty that can lead nowhere because he is unable to commit himself to anyone other than Nicole. Having given too much of himself in his self-interested ministering to her, Diver, once she is healed, is reminiscent of the fiendish Roger Chillingworth who withers once Dimmesdale, his maligned patient, begins to recover.

Unable to survive Nicole's recovery, Dick Diver fades away, all but disappearing as he returns to upstate New York where he continues to practice medicine. He, who had once traveled the Continent in "fabulous" style, drifts from Buffalo to Batavia to Lockport. "He was considered to have fine manners and once made a good speech at a public health meeting on the subject of drugs; but he became entangled with a girl who worked in a grocery store, and he was also involved in a lawsuit about some medical question; so he left Lockport." From there he goes on to Geneva, then to Hornell, and in the narrator's final comment, there is no question but that Dick Diver is lost: "In any case he is almost certainly in that section of the country, in one town or another" (p. 344).

Equally lost and for much the same self-centered reason is Harry Wilbourne, the intern-protagonist of William Faulkner's *The Wild Palms* (1939).[15] Another inversion of the idealized doctor, Wilbourne in his lack of self-knowledge is similar to Dick Diver, and in his unsuitability for a medical career he is another echo of S. Weir Mitchell's Dr. Ezra Wendell. Like Diver, too, Wilbourne is ironically named since he is neither well born (his father was a poor country doctor) nor able to bear up well in face of the world around him. This inability to face and cope with life is the focus of the novel and the underlying cause of Wilbourne's decline.

Startlingly uncommitted to his chosen profession, Wilbourne, who awakens on the morning of his twenty-seventh birthday and looks at those years "as if his life were to lie passively on his back as he floated effortless and without volition on an unreturning stream" (pp. 33–34), sees medicine as a series of empty routines to be performed in order to maintain his detachment from life and people. Like Anderson's Dr. Parcival, Wilbourne is a doctor (in training) who does not really want nor care about patients. Into his uncaring routines bursts the vibrant Charlotte Rittenmeyer, unhappily married and filled with an anarchic zest for life. She penetrates his carefully constructed shell of self-isolating medical activity, takes him as her lover, and persuades him to leave New Orleans with her.

Desiring to escape the world's dullness through passion, Charlotte finds that she can escape only into another form of Wilbourne's frozen isolation. Having said to him, " 'It's got to be all honeymoon, always . . . Either heaven or hell: no safe comfortable purgatory' " (p. 83), she soon discovers that she is trapped in a purgatory of banality. No more able to commit himself to Charlotte than he'd been able to commit himself to medicine or to patients or to any portion of life around him, Wilbourne, once removed from the safe routines of internship, is set adrift as he and Charlotte go from Chicago to a Wisconson lakeside town, then on to a Utah mining camp, and finally to a small Mississippi coastal village.

Once there, Charlotte persuades Wilbourne to perform an abortion on her since she fears that the intrusion of even a wanted child will destroy totally the small seed of rebellious love that ties them together. Yet Wilbourne, once enamored of the safety of medical routine, botches the routine abortion, not because he lacks skill but because he cannot bear the consequences of succeeding, namely a continuation of his life with Charlotte.

The outcome of his final withdrawal is complete isolation and self-destruction. Charlotte dies, and Wilbourne is arrested, tried, convicted, and sentenced to fifty years at hard labor (p. 321). Given the means to commit suicide by Charlotte's distraught husband, Wilbourne refuses, preferring the safe routines of prison to the final negation and uncertainty of death, saying to himself, " 'Yes . . . between grief and nothing I will take grief' " (p. 324). Thus consigning himself to oblivion, Wilbourne, like Steinbeck's Doc Burton and Fitzgerald's Dick Diver, disappears from the world he can neither see clearly nor accept fully. Having violated the prime tenet of his profession by killing his wife and their unborn child, Wilbourne, the personification of the anti-ideal, sinks at last into a "grief" that will shield him at last from the world that he cannot bear.

Faulkner, then, like other of America's best writers from Hawthorne on, creates in Wilbourne a doctor far different from the idealized type more often presented to the American reading public. Working to achieve particular thematic ends, Faulkner capitalizes on the evocative nature of the fictionalized ideal by setting his own far-from-ideal intern against an already familiar and well-known type. Harry Wilbourne, who lacks will, compassion, and self-knowledge, appears even more lacking when juxtaposed against the collective idealization. Thus the benevolent actions and admirable characteristics of Wilbourne's fictional predecessors (from Holmes's good Dr. Kittredge through James's clear-eyed Sir Luke Strett) stand in silent condemnation of his own destructive actions.

AMERICA'S BEST-SELLING DOCTORS AND DOCTOR-PRIESTS

The negative judgment that a reader passes on Harry Wilbourne is intensified by what has come to be expected of doctors in their fictional worlds and in actual life. Judged against the collective ideal, Wilbourne, like Ezra Wendell before him, is found lacking, but unlike Wendell, Harry Wilbourne can be seen within a larger context, one that goes beyond the particular world of medicine and resonates with the experiences of all people's lives.

As do other fine American writers, Faulkner subordinates his fictional doctor within a complex rendering of particular thematic concerns. This thematic use of the doctor (in either the ideal form or in its antithesis) demonstrates a fundamental difference between literary "art" and popular literature. Literature that is art is timeless and presents characters involved in generalizable situations. In contrast, popular literature is time-bound and presents characters who function in highly particularized fictional worlds. Popular literature captures the here and now of a particular time and place and rarely goes beyond that, whereas literary art, although it may capture the essence of a certain time and place, does so only in the service of more complex ends.

This distinction is evident in the novels that have come to be known as "best-sellers," a term that came into existence in 1895 when *The Bookman* began compiling (for the use of book sellers) America's first comprehensive lists of book sales.[16] Since that time seven medical novels—*The Doctor* (Connor), *Main Street, Arrowsmith, Magnificent Obsession, The Doctor,* (Rinehart), *Not As A Stranger, Testimony of Two Men*—have been, in hardbound editions, annual best-sellers, (*Magnificent Obsession* and *Not As A Stranger* appeared on the list in two consecutive years.) In addition, three others—*Spencer Brade, M.D., The Interns,* and *The Wild Palms*—attained paperback sales of over one-million copies, sufficient to be denoted paperback best-sellers.[17]

Although there are criteria other than Hackett's by which to determine "best-seller" status[18] and there is no clear agreement about whether a best-seller "formula" really exists,[19] there is good reason to believe that books popular enough to become known as best-sellers are of use in attempting to understand a people's ways of doing things. In *The Popular Book,* James

D. Hart maintains that rather than the "classics," it is the popular books that yield more for the student of a particular period since "books flourish when they answer a need and die when they do not." Hart, however, is not content with easy generalizations and cautions that any conclusions about the causes of a book's popularity must account for the "dynamic interplay of reader, writer, and the times in which both lived."[20] That cultural interplay must be kept continually in mind while examining the varied writings that have contributed to the making of America's medical myth. As it is embodied in the best-selling novels of the past eighty years, despite substantial change within the medical profession and among the American reading public, the myth of the doctor-priest has retained its potency and basic characteristics to a remarkable degree.

Exemplary of the kind of best-seller that is time-bound and that exhibits only limited appeal beyond the years immediately following its publication is Ralph Connor's 1906 novel *The Doctor*, which ranked ninth on the 1907 best-seller list. The title character is Barney Boyle, the "born doctor,"[21] who decides to sacrifice his own ambition so that his brother, Dick, may study for the ministry. But Barney, whose jaw and chin "suggested the bed rock of character, abiding, firm, indomitable" (p. 66), has sufficient intensity of purpose to know that he will somehow become a doctor. Barney Boyle is aided in his resolve by the good and aging Dr. Ferguson, who advises him, lends him books, and remains the young man's supporter even when Boyle twice fails his medical exams (p. 114). Anxious to arouse maximum reader interest, Connor also adds a romantic subplot in the form of a triangle composed of Barney, his brother, and Barney's beloved Iola, whom he loses, first to her ambition for a singing career (p. 161) and then to his brother, who has failed his ministerial exams and becomes a journalist while Barney finishes medical school and is appointed to the staff of Johns Hopkins Hospital (p. 177). In despair at losing Iola, Barney flees to Europe, fights death in the form of a diptheria epidemic (p. 244), and upon his return to America, becomes medical superintendent for a railroad construction camp (p. 272).

While Barney is soothing his broken heart in a flurry of work, Dick, finally succeeding in the ministry, brings Iola, sick and still in love with Barney, back from Europe. Connor thickens his plot by having Barney begrudgingly save his brother's life and finally forgive him upon learning that the dying Iola still loves him (Barney) as she did before their separation. Barney, strong in both his chosen profession and in his love for Iola, grows even stronger as he becomes, literally, a doctor-priest who will preach in his brother's place as Dick convalesces.

Barney's happiness is short-lived, however, and upon Iola's death (p. 360), the poker-playing doctor-priest repudiates his amoral ways and uses his poker winnings for the common good by installing libraries and clubrooms in the railroad construction camps. "To his former care for the physical well-being of the men, he added now a concern for their mental and spiritual good" (p. 379). Having thus become the altruistic doctor-priest, there is nothing more that Barney Boyle can do (given his creator's penchant for melodrama) but die in the service of the sick and needy.

In the melodramatic and didactic conclusion, Connor mounts a monumental funeral cortege that will return the good doctor to his final resting place:

> Two thousand miles and more they carried him home to his mother, and then to the old churchyard, where he sleeps still, forgotten, perhaps even by many who had known and played with him in his boyhood, but remembered by the men of the mountains who had once felt the touch of that strong love that gave the best and freely for their sakes, and for His Whom it was his pride and joy to call Master and Friend. (p. 396)

Having evolved, while alive, from a poker-playing doctor to a preaching doctor-priest, Barney Boyle in death is even further elevated to the status of "Friend" of the "Master" if not to actual sainthood. Working with already familiar materials, Connor gives his readers an exaggerated if not memorable example of the growing idealization.

Far different in tone and quality from Connor's melodramatic pastiche are the two medical novels of Pulitzer and Nobel prizewinner Sinclair Lewis, novels that handle familiar material both well and thoroughly. Of these, *Main Street*, first on the 1921 best-seller list, casts as a background figure its country doctor Will Kennicott in order to focus on the dilemma and growth of his wife, Carol, a woman who wants a richer, more rewarding life.[22] Reminiscent of Elizabeth Willard in *Winesburg, Ohio*, Carol Milford Kennicott, a graduate of Blodgett College, determines to earn her own living, spends a year in Chicago, then goes on to work in the St. Paul Public Library (p. 16). After three uninspiring years, she meets Dr. Will Kennicott, they fall in love, and she finally consents to marry him and go to Gopher Prairie, one more of that endless stream of planless midwestern towns. Jolted from her naive dreams of improving the town, Carol quickly realizes that Gopher Prairie is merely a variant of all the small towns she has known. Only to the eyes of a Kennicott was it exceptional (p. 30). Worse still, she realizes that she is trapped.

The nature of the trap and her reactions to it undergird the novel's plot, a crucial part being the slow growth of Carol's admiration for her husband. Will Kennicott, devoted to making money and realistic in his self-assessment about becoming case-hardened (pp. 19–21), seems initially to be the antithesis of the ideal doctor. In the first four chapters, tightly focused through Carol's eyes, there is virtually nothing seen of Kennicott's doctoring. Only when he takes her off to the country for a day of hunting that allows her to break free from the torpor of Gopher Prairie does Carol (and the reader) have a chance at a more complete view of Dr. Will Kennicott. In the admiration for him shown by one of his patients whom they encounter on their outing, Carol sees a side of her husband she barely recognizes, and in her characteristic zeal she exaggerates the reality, heightening and romanticizing it (p. 59).

Unable to accept Will Kennicott and Gopher Prairie for what they are, Carol unwittingly distorts them, both overestimating and debasing their reality, and in doing so subverts her own best intentions to reform her small world. Typical of her blithe disregard for others is her decision to redecorate Kennicott's house. She throws away the old furniture, and, although wanting to idealize her doctor-husband, unthinkingly discards Fildes's portrait, *The Doctor* (p. 70), the quintessential visualization of the ideal country physician, showing "a hovel, a sick child, a group of anxious parents, and as its central figure, a glossy-bearded [doctor leaning] over the dying innocent."[23]

The disparity between the idealization depicted in the painting and the reality that Carol perceives in her mundane doctor-husband echoes the disparity between the world she dreams of and the one she finds in Gopher Prairie where she discovers that she has nothing to do but become Dr. Kennicott's wife. As that change occurs, Carol Kennicott grows up, and in growing she becomes more aware of the true and deeper nature of the town. Her coming to awareness covers the bulk of the novel, a crucial element of which is an increasingly complex and sympathetic view of Will Kennicott, far more realistic than the view in Fildes's painting, yet one that shares in and contributes its own ambience to the evolving idealization of the American physician.

The change in Carol Kennicott's attitude toward her husband, a parallel to her evolving view of herself and the larger world around her, takes place slowly, and in a manner typical of Lewis's ironic fiction, it is often undercut. Beginning to admire Will as she learns how much his patients regard him, she generalizes her admiration and argues with a friend that medicine shouldn't be and isn't a business. Carol, who wants to believe that all doctors—and therefore her husband—are priestly and selfless healers (as did many of Lewis's readers), is unable to accept the fact that fallibility and less-than-admirable traits are as likely to be a part of doctors as of any other people.

In contrast to Carol's exaggerated idealizations is the level-headed and good-natured view of his colleagues that Will holds. He admits that there are rivalries among Gopher Prairie's doctors and that their competence is often less than it appears to their patients (pp. 161–165). Yet even these declarations of truth about his world do not temper Carol's impulse to idealize her husband as a healer, an impulse rendered by Lewis with sympathetic irony when Carol must assist Will to amputate a German farmer's arm. In the midst of seeping blood, choking ether fumes, and surgical necessity, Carol comes to see her husband in a different light.

What she actually sees is depicted by Lewis as carefully as *The Doctor* had been painted by Fildes. Fighting nausea, Carol stumbles outside for air, then returns to her task:

> As she returned she caught the scene as a whole . . . in the center, illuminated by a small glass lamp held by a frightened stout woman, Dr. Kennicott [was] bending over a body which was humped under a sheet—the oxygen, his bare arms daubed with blood, his hands . . . loosening the tourniquet, his face without emotion save when he threw up his head and chuckled at the farmwife, "Hold that light steady just a second more—*noch blos ein wenig.*" (p. 188)

For Carol (and for the reader), this sharply etched scene reveals Will Kennicott at his best and most competent, and Lewis, well in control of his ironic presentation, moves swiftly from the objective scene back into Carol's response to it, a response that exhibits both her heightened awareness and her inevitable tendency to romanticize the world: " 'He speaks a vulgar, common incorrect German of life and death and birth and the soil. I read the French and German of sentimental lovers and Christmas garlands. And I thought that it was I who had the culture!' " (p. 188) she thinks worshipfully.

In awe of Will for what he can do under stress, Carol finds that awe cannot be sustained in their daily life. She feels more and more trapped by the unyielding dreariness of Gopher Prairie and is forced to admit to herself that she has been trying to do the impossible. Increasingly enfeebled by loneliness, in her frustration she comes to view Will as an enemy to whom she is yoked. In turn, feeling more and more estranged from his wife, Will embarks on an affair with one of his patients while Carol takes up with Erick Valborg, a young tailor who offends the townspeople with his effete refinements.

Aware of Gopher Prairie's disapproval of Carol's flirtation, Will, in an attempt to warn her that the town will have its revenge, speaks of himself and of his love for her in a scene that is an evocative self-portrait of the small-town doctor:

> "Now it's my turn [he says] . . . Carrie, do you understand my work? . . . No matter even if you are cold, I like you better than anybody in the world. One time I said that you were my soul. And that still goes . . . Do you realize what my job is? I go round twenty-four hours a day . . . trying my damnedest to heal everybody, rich or poor. . . . And I can stand the cold and the bumpy roads and the lonely rides at night. All I need is to have you here at home to welcome me. I don't expect you to be passionate—not any more I don't—but I do expect you to appreciate my work." (p. 381)

Here, the personal and professional worlds of Will Kennicott merge, and the reader is able to see a whole man, skilled and dedicated, yet not without flaws. Unfortunately, this view is not shared by the doctor's wife. Shaken by the realization that Valborg will not be her means to escape from Gopher Prairie's dreariness and aware that she cannot, finally, leave Will or escape her stultifying life, she persuades him to take her to California for a three-month respite. Once back home, after actually becoming anxious to return, Carol is soon appalled and decides that she must leave so that she can have the time to discover what she wants (p. 405).

After moving to Washington, D.C., she discovers at first that the freedom she has attained is empty, that the long-coveted job she has won is boring, that an urban office can be as petty as Gopher Prairie. Yet faced with this new disillusioning reality, she comes to grips with her world for the first time in her life, and she begins to feel the strength that comes from her growing autonomy.

In Washington she discovers many of Main Street's worst flaws, but in her growing maturity she is newly able to accept the world on its own terms and to come to a clearer understanding and fuller appreciation of Will.

Strengthened by her time alone and finally aware that she no longer hates Gopher Prairie, Carol decides to return to her husband. The novel's closing scene presents a final exchange between Dr. Kennicott and his wiser-though-still-and-forever-enthusiastic wife, an exchange that shows clearly that Will Kennicott, skilled and limited as he is, will prevail, that the mundane—whether rightly or wrongly—will triumph simply by being able to endure:

> "I've never excused my failures by sneering at my aspirations," [said Carol,] "by pretending to have gone beyond them . . . I may not have fought the good fight, but I have kept the faith."
> "Sure. You bet you have," said Kennicott. "Well, good night . . . Have to be thinking about putting up the storm windows pretty soon. Say, did you notice whether the girl put that screw-driver back?" (p. 432)

Focused on, and largely through, the perceptions of Carol Kennicott, *Main Street* partakes of crucial elements of America's evolving medical myth. Lewis, although willing to chuckle at Will Kennicott's foibles (and those of all the others in the novel), is sympathetic toward the small-town doctor. That underlying sympathy is the very thing that permits a reader also to chuckle at and, in turn, appreciate Kennicott.

A kindred sympathy and the clarity of vision it allows are also central to Lewis's successful creation, five years later, of a far different kind of doctor in *Arrowsmith*, the number seven best-seller in 1925. The sympathetic underpinnings of both novels are understandable in light of the fact that Lewis's father, grandfather, older brother, and uncle were doctors. When in 1922 he was persuaded by a friend, Dr. Morris Fishbein, and by bacteriologist Paul de Kruif to begin work on a novel about medical research, Lewis's own vicarious medical experience served him well. For the more technical and detailed materials, he hired de Kruif, who educated him in bacteriology and epidemiology and provided considerable source material for *Arrowsmith's* medical world.[24]

Atypical of its genre in having a wealth of primary characters forming a microcosm of the medical profession, the novel also differs from its predecessors in the way it moves its title character, Martin Arrowsmith, from medical school on through larger and more complex medical spheres. Arrowsmith, whom the ironic narrator early describes as "a young man who was in no degree a hero, who regarded himself as a seeker after truth yet who stumbled and slid back all his life and bogged himself down in every obvious morass,"[25] is far different from the staunchly individualistic doctors of good character whose benevolent actions lent substance to the collective idealization of which they were a part.

Martin Arrowsmith, in his journey toward self-actualization as a true doctor-scientist, functions at all times within a highly structured and often adversarial profession. In his quest "for the causes of things" (p. 108), he tries his hand at being a country G. P., a public health doctor, a member of a wealthy Chicago clinic, and a researcher for a prestigious scientific institute. At each stage of his career, though, he prefers the "barbarian loneliness" (p. 33) that had come to be his mode in medical school when he first worked with and embarked on the path of pure science under the guidance of Max Gottlieb.

Even Gottlieb, the single most influential person in Arrowsmith's life, is put aside as are all the rest of the young doctor's heroes so that he can become the dedicated scientist he is destined to become. Although able to enact the necessary metaphoric slayings of his various heroes, Arrowsmith has more difficulty slaying once and for all the larger forces that threaten his dedication to medical science—namely success, crass commercialism, and the materialism that those engender and that continually attracts him. Yet even those forces and their persuasive representatives are finally transcended in Arrowsmith's quest for pure, scientific truth, a quest whose intensity and consequences turn him into a doctor-scientist who, by caring "infinitely more for science than for mankind," is an ironic echo of Hawthorne's arch-fiend Rappaccini. Suffering defeat and embarrassment, risking fame and spurning fortune, losing one wife to an epidemic he is fighting and another to the research into which her wealthy life cannot fit, Arrowsmith is intensely individualistic, self-centered, and ever more obsessed (as was Rappaccini) with learning the true causes of things.

Doing much the same thing that Rappaccini had done, Arrowsmith is, nevertheless, cast in an heroic mold, despite the narrator's earlier and ironic remarks to the contrary. The fact that Lewis chooses to make his isolated man of science a hero rather than an arch-fiend is one indicator of how, in the three-quarters of a century separating Hawthorne and Lewis, American attitudes toward science had changed. Once mistrusted and little understood, science had by the 1920s become familiar and beneficent enough to seem trustworthy. Only when science had thus been tamed in the public mind could the singleminded doctor-scientist do his work in an heroic rather than a demonic mode. Even the good character and beneficent concern for others that characterize Arrowsmith's fictional predecessors can be laid aside without their absence seriously damaging Lewis's honorific portrait. Ostensibly far different from doctors Kittredge, North, Leslie, Strett, and others, Martin Arrowsmith is, on the more fundamental level of public need and desire, their direct descendent.

Having retreated to the Vermont woods with his colleague Terry Wickett in order to be free from the world of patients and emotional involvement so that he can dedicate himself to research, Arrowsmith becomes a man reborn:

> His mathematics and physical chemistry were now as sound as Terry's, his indifference to publicity and to flowery hangings as great, his industry as fanatical, his ingenuity in devising new apparatus at least comparable, and his imagination far more swift. He had less ease but more passion. He hurled out hypotheses like sparks. He began, incredulously, to comprehend his freedom. He would yet determine the essential nature of phage; and as he became stronger and surer—and no doubt less human—he saw ahead of him innumerous inquiries into chemotherapy and immunity; enough adventures to keep him busy for decades. (p. 428)

In his single-minded dedication, in his refusal to compromise with a society more concerned with titles than with test tubes, Arrowsmith retains the aura of sanctity of a beneficient priest in the temple of science. When last seen, Arrowsmith and Terry Wickett are together, lolling "in a clumsy boat, an extraordinarily uncomfortable boat, far out on" their Vermont lake. In a final gesture that characterizes his hero as a doctor-scientist working for the good of all people, Lewis gives Arrowsmith a concluding speech that indicates that the "barbarian's" dedicated quest for the "causes of things" has not blinded him to his own human fallibility or to the need for a willingness to start ever anew: "I feel as if I were really beginning to work now," said Martin. "This new quinine stuff may prove pretty good. We'll plug along on it for two or three years, and maybe we'll get something permanent—and probably we'll fail!" (p. 430).

Since *Arrowsmith*, there has been no medical novel of comparable quality, although the genre has continued to spawn best-sellers, some of whose total sales have exceeded those of Lewis's novel. Distinguished less for its literary merit than for the fact that it has sold nearly three million copies (in combined hard and paper-bound editions)[26] is Lloyd C. Douglas's *Magnificent Obsession*, first published in 1929, which placed eighth on the 1932 best-seller list and moved up to fourth place the following year.

Joining as it does medical myth with a religious tract enlivened by a melodramatic love story, the novel found a ready audience that grew steadily during the first half-decade following publication. *Book Review Digest* summarized it succinctly:

> The "magnificent obsession" that was the secret of the famous Dr. Hudson's success—a newly interpreted Christian teaching—was put into practice at Dr. Hudson's death by the young man who became his successor as a brain surgeon, Bobby Merrick. Bobby, by continuing his "personality investments" in the way of secret philanthropies, as advocated by Dr. Hudson's formula, miraculously succeeds, and makes a famous surgical invention with which he is able to save the life of the woman he loves.[27]

Within the framework of his often astounding plot, Douglas, himself a retired minister, adds embellishments that overburden an already implausible tale with melodramatic trappings that likely contributed to the book's popularity. Bobby Merrick, whose life is saved by the very inhalator needed to keep Dr. Hudson alive, is shocked out of his playboy life when he learns that he had been inadvertently responsible for the famous brain surgeon's death. Merrick decides that he will become a surgeon, and he gains possession of the cryptic journal, which, once its code is broken, yields the secret of Hudson's magnificent obsession and consequent success.

As Merrick thrives by putting into practice Hudson's precepts about aiding the needy and then using their personalities to improve his own, he becomes embroiled in an unlikely romantic triangle, loved by Hudson's daughter, Joyce, and himself in love with Hudson's widow, Helen. Rejected by the woman he loves and having experienced a mystical conversion after lending $5,000 to a fellow medical student, Merrick throws himself totally into his work.[28]

With what Douglas clearly intends to be taken as the intervention of God, Merrick invents a self-cauterizing scalpel that will "completely revolutionize brain surgery and make a new science of it" (p. 199). Not content to leave Merrick alone with his dedication and success, Douglas takes the last third of the novel to resolve the brilliant young surgeon's romantic difficulties and to devise an appropriately contrived ending.

Unable, however, to sustain the medical, religious, and philanthropic strains, Douglas falls back onto the hackneyed boy pursues, loses, pursues, gets girl scenario. Helen Hudson, having fled to Europe to work after learning that Merrick's philanthropy has also benefitted her, is critically injured in a train wreck and loses her sight (p. 266). Merrick rushes to her bedside and decides that he must face the risks involved and operate. With expectable success, he restores her sight (p. 272) and attempts to keep his identity and achievement a secret so that his beloved will not feel further indebted to him.

Finally, love triumphs and Merrick and Helen Hudson, now able to see him for the dedicated and good man he has become, are married (p. 282). Thus the playboy, reformed by the teachings of Dr. Hudson's secret obsession, takes on the mantle of priestlike philanthropy, projects the strength of his personality into others in dire need, and is finally rewarded with the love of the woman he had, inadvertently, made a widow.

Contrived though it is, Douglas' novel is more readable and was understandably far more popular than the number nine best-seller of 1935, Mary Roberts Rinehart's *The Doctor*. Herself a doctor's wife and a nursing school graduate (she had wanted to be a doctor), Rinehart makes much use of personal experience in her elaborately plotted medical romance. Yet the novel often seems to be written by someone with little firsthand knowledge of the medical world, a fact that Rinehart, in her autobiography, accounts for when she explains her own reticence about capitalizing on the experiences she had been privy to, saying that since she was not a realist she "did not want to recall them."[29] Another statement in the autobiography, to explain how she calculatedly tried to strengthen her early fiction, also helps to explain the loose, often implausible plotting of *The Doctor*. She writes, "To bolster my faulty craftsmanship, I resorted to plot, that crutch of the beginner, that vice of the experienced writer. I devised weird and often horrible plots. I could think faster than I could write, devise plots and put them on paper with amazing speed" (p. 86).

Although written half a decade after those remarks were recorded, *The Doctor* exemplifies the kind of plotting that Rinehart labels both "crutch" and "vice." Focused on the career of Dr. Chris Arden, the novel is a pastiche of familiar elements. Arden, first introduced as a disheveled young resident, upon reaching the hospital ward, becomes a "King. More, he would be a god of a sort; nurses hurrying to obey his orders ... and watching him with interest, and perhaps some feeble life hanging on his quickness, his skill."[30]

Like many of his fictional predecessors, Chris Arden had been influenced by a country doctor, old Dave Mortimer, who according to his friends saved lives "as though he were fighting death by sheer will power" (p. 17). So influenced, Arden chooses to begin his career as a small-town doctor, and though he is aided by the influence of his wealthy friends, he is enough of an independent spirit to announce that the typhoid epidemic is the responsibility of one of the town's leading citizens (p. 52). Having early established her hero's willingness to confront the local power structure, Rinehart moves quickly to drive home the point that the individualistic young doctor, though overburdened with patients, understands their need for a priestly healer:

> This was his apprenticeship, and already he knew that; men or women, often what they wanted was something more than drugs and care ... the real moment came for them when, having put away thermometer and watch, he sat back in his chair beside the bed ... This was their hour, the one time when as to a priest they poured out their anxieties and griefs, and even their sins ...

> They wanted reassurance as well as confession. They wanted forgiveness. By some metonymy their doctors became to them almost a symbol of deity, and their confessions were like prayers. (pp. 99–100)

Concerned and skilled though he is, it is inevitable, given the plot, that Arden should confront failure via the death of one of his patients. Just as inevitable is the advice given to him to an older colleague, Dr. Grant, who says, " 'We can't be gods ... we are only men, so we have to draw a balance ... You'll always save more than you lose; but you will always have losses. Better think of them as cases, not as men and women. Then you can carry on' " (p. 205). Grant's advice here is an example of what Talcott Parsons describes as "affective neutrality," the ability of doctors to maintain a degree of detachment sufficient to allow them to treat a patient without becoming overly involved emotionally and, hence, less effective.[31]

Antithetical as it is to the well-established fictional tradition of the doctor as benevolent and concerned healer, Dr. Grant's advice is also antithetical to the best interests of Chris Arden, whose practice flourishes and who finds it all too easy to regard more and more of the people he treats as just cases. Having lost the delicate balance between the right degree of necessary detachment and equally necessary concern, Arden, more and more successful, finds himself burned out; he discovers that he has become cool, competent, and efficient, a money-making machine with little heart and no passion for the healing he once loved.

The decline, self-renewal, and eventual recovery of Arden provide the major unifying force to Rinehart's novel, but her own admitted penchant for writing romances leads her to bring about that recovery by means of a romantic subplot, which repeatedly eclipses the novel's main concerns. Unhappy with his successful but increasingly hollow career and burdened with an unhappy marriage, Arden, in keeping with Rinehart's preference for "weird and often horrible plots," is a prime target for "catastrophe" (*My Story*, p. 420), which comes in the form of an automobile accident that cuts the "musculo-spiral nerve," leaving him in a condition where "only Providence could save him from a useless arm" (p. 429).

The providential recovery comes in predictable stages, beginning with Arden's decision to leave his lucrative practice and return to his hometown to search out the pattern of his life (p. 416). Relieved by his wife's final willingness to divorce him, the despairing doctor successfully battles alcoholism and is given the chance at last to begin his return to medicine when he is called to a nearby bedside: "He spent most of that night by the child's bed in a small village house, content to be there, to hear the long crowing intake of air grow less stertorous. Once more—small as it was—he made a fight and won it ... He was still needed, could still be useful" (pp. 466–67).

Alluding, as she clearly does here, to Fildes' highly romanticized painting of *The Doctor*, Rinehart goes on to devise a final melodramatic stage to Chris Arden's recovery and transformation into still another familiar and ideal "good" doctor. Having again become a country doctor, Arden, long and frustratedly in love with Beverly Lewis, learns that she is in need of surgery that she wants him to perform. With feeling beginning to return to his damaged arm and with the confidence gained by having successfully operated on his foster son, Arden goes to Beverly as she is undergoing surgery for a perforated ulcer. Unable to help the woman he desperately loves, Arden finds himself "an onlooker, useless" (p. 502), and realizing fully his desperate need to be wholly functional again, he undergoes the final stage of his recovery. Quite conveniently, his beloved Beverly enjoys a rapid recovery, and as Arden stays with her at the hospital, he is asked by the house surgeon to advise on another case.

Having returned to and been accepted by the medical world he had lost, Dr. Chris Arden re-enters the operating room in triumph: "They moved aside for him, and now he was there once more, where he belonged. Instantly he was absorbed, intent. The past was wiped away, even the present. All that existed for him at that moment was the case before him" (p. 506). A wiser and more compassionate man for what he has learned from his suffering, Chris Arden can return to the surgery he loves, and he can regain the balance that allows him the necessary professional detachment to view his patients as cases without becoming hardened to their needs as people. Akin to Martin Arrowsmith, whose zealous dedication to scientific research is admirable because it is directed to humane ends, Chris Arden's total involvement with his surgical skill remains laudable because it has been tempered by the experiences (melodramatic as they are) that have humanized and made him a true healer.

Nearly two decades later, the same concern for the humanization of an isolated and uncaring though otherwise skilled doctor formed the basis for 1954's number-one best-seller, Morton Thompson's *Not As A Stranger* (which dropped to seventh place on the 1955 best-seller list). Among the most well written of the best-selling medical novels, Thompson's book is a model rendering of those elements most basic to the medical myth that had been evolving for nearly a full century.

Taking its title from *Job* 19:26–27 (". . . yet in my flesh shall I see God:/ whom I shall see for myself,/ and mine eyes shall behold him,/ and not as a stranger"), the novel follows the career of Lucas Marsh, a doctor-priest who, through his experiences and suffering, comes (as Job had come to see God) to a clear view of himself and his profession.

Even as a child, Marsh was enamored of the local doctors' world,[32] and by the age of seven, after the accidental death of his pet chick and his ministering to the town's flea-infested dogs, he knew that he wanted to be a doctor. Possessing the intensity of purpose characteristic of the best of his fictional precursors, young Marsh overcomes his father's adamant objections and the family's financial difficulties to enter medical school. Achieving his goal, he becomes an ecstatic neophyte, a medical student whose view of his chosen profession is cast repeatedly in religious terms: "He came into the hospital . . . [and] looked about him, acolyte-hungry, and all about him was the incense of the temple, the smell of formaldehyde . . . and a hundred other chemicals" (p. 137).

The religious view, however, is not Marsh's alone; the third-person narrator draws back and describes the new acolyte in similar language: "It was not . . . a young man standing there . . . It was spirit, the inner drive of man . . . and this stood waiting for the vessel of flesh in which it was contained to carry it forward to the world in which it could be God" (p. 137). This direct evocation of the doctor as God foreshadows the novel's central plot, which traces Lucas Marsh's career throughout the years in which he changes from a dedicated student into an angry and isolated physician and finally into a humane doctor-priest, a true successor of his Biblical namesake Luke, the beloved physician. That Marsh will, after his long initiation and apprenticeship, become a true and beloved physician is hinted at early in the novel when he witnesses his first operation and is jolted from the detachment of the new medical student: " . . . suddenly Lucas had seen the whole patient . . . This was a whole human being. The impact shattered his objectivity, projected him onto the table" (p. 238).

The empathy that Marsh feels is matched by his intense desire to become a doctor, a desire that allows nothing to stand in its way and drives him to fulfill his vow, to do anything to succeed. Left penniless by his father's bankruptcy, Marsh, who has already attached himself to the operating room's charge nurse Kristina Hedvigsen in order to gain access to the OR, decides to marry her in order to gain the financial security that will allow him to continue his studies. Fully aware that his plan is wrong and willing to steal if it should fail, Marsh, in his desperation to continue his studies, understands that for him there are no longer rules. There is only necessity (pp. 286–287).

That necessity, actualized in his intense drive, helps Marsh cope with the rigors of medical school that begin almost immediately on his first day when he sees that his natural aloofness cannot serve him well. He and his fellow students realize that they must learn to cooperate in spite of their differences. As they cling together, they fall into a pattern so characteristic of the realities of medical education that the novel can well be read as a case history for Becker's 1961 study of medical school socialization, *Boys in White*.

Part of that pattern is competition in class balanced outside of class by mutual support. This help is needed because initially Marsh, the typical medical student, is swamped with work. What he must learn is how to decide what to learn, and that crucial first lesson is fast and well absorbed. Having established what Becker would come to call (more than half a decade after Thompson's novel) the "provisional perspective,"[33] Marsh learns an even more crucial fact of medical life when he realizes that the inevitability of incompetent doctors, lacking dedication and concern, can neither harm him nor damage the profession he has chosen. Realizing this, he is able, grimly, to tolerate the imperfections of others, all the while disdaining them. The disdain that Marsh feels for these "interlopers" he soon comes to feel for the very patients he treats. By the time he is an intern, patients for Marsh are only a means to a far greater end—medicine—to which he devotes his entire being, working intensely and feeling nothing but contempt for anything that interrupts his pursuit.

Among the unwanted interruptions are the materialistic attitudes that Marsh finds among his colleagues and at which he rails. Juxtaposed against his vehement idealism are the more realistic views of Dr. Aarons, one of his professors, and of Avery, a fellow student. After one of Marsh's outbursts against the stupidity of some doctors, Aarons says sharply, " 'It is very clear that what you want is a shrine, some great and famous Lourdes where you can worship, tended by priests world-known for their piety, their integrity and their glory' " (p. 365).

Even more pointed are the cynical remarks of Avery, who becomes increasingly impatient with Marsh and who tries repeatedly to make the hopelessly idealistic intern see how unattainable are the expectations he holds for himself and for his profession. In one of his tirades, Avery speaks of the public's awe of its doctors:

> "And do you know what holds us together?[he asks.] Our union? It's fear and ignorance. To the average human his body is a great and sacred mystery. And the man who knows the riddle of the mystery is a god. That's what we are—gods. And the thing that holds us together as a group is our realization of this. We know how the public feels about us." (p. 373)

Clearly anxious to capitalize on the contrast between Marsh and Avery, Thompson has the latter continue his diatribe in terms that repeatedly draw upon the tradition of the benevolent and priestly doctor. Though willing to grant that some doctors are dedicated and selfless, Avery maintains that most are neither, and he complains bitterly about the phenomenon of professional solidarity and the consequent tendency to encourage people's misperceptions: " 'Not the fact [he says] that they think we're witch doctors. That's terrible enough. But the way we encourage them to think that way' " (p. 374).

Committed to an ideal of medical infallibility, Marsh is impervious to these criticisms, and he is unable to recognize the truth of his friend's words when Avery accuses him of lacking genuine concern for patients and of regarding them less as people than as the materials of his art (p. 375). In his desire to join the medical priesthood, Marsh loses sight of the people he will heal, regards them as no more than materials for his use, and comes finally to disdain them just as he disdains the incompetents who defile the temple of healers. Marsh is as blind to life and to the human truth of medicine as Job was to the reasons for his suffering, and like Job, Marsh also becomes "an alien in [others] sight" (*Job* 19:15) before he can begin the transformation that will turn him, by the novel's end, into a true and compassionate healer. Finished with medical school, Marsh takes his first job as assistant to Dr. Runkleman, a backwoods surgeon whom he comes quickly to admire. After his first day with patients, the new doctor loses all traces of uncertainty; "he was all that he had learned, he was an instrument" (p. 447).

Marsh evolves from doctor-in-training to doctor-as-instrument—cool, efficient, detached—always ready and able to heal others, never able to feel for or with them. Admiring Runkleman while isolating himself more and more in his own work, raging at his growing disillusionment with his colleagues' materialism (p. 524) while he fears that he, too, is being corrupted and forced to conform, Marsh is even disabused (by Avery) of any notion that by turning to teaching he might escape the sullying of his medical temple. Out of his rage and frustrations grows a new and dangerous resolve: He would treat as many patients as well as he could; quantity would yield quality care. Substituting quantity of contact for the unattained quality of genuine relationship with any of his patients, Marsh loses all ability to see those he treats as anything more than cases and symptoms.

Blind to all but his own desires and isolated so totally that an exasperated colleague calls him "a stranger to the world" (p. 269), Marsh must, as had both his own father and his father's Biblical namesake, Job, suffer so that he, too, may learn. Only through suffering—through the loss of Runkleman, through the near dissolution of his marriage, through the agonies of a typhoid epidemic, and through the painful realization that his profession is, in fact, a genuine priesthood that "did not try [its members] for murder [but only] for heresy...did not execute...[but] protected its own" (p. 882)—only through all of these experiences does Marsh begin to learn that medicine is not his alone but belongs to all of his colleagues (p. 885) and that he must give up his splendid isolation and the maniacal and destructive belief that once the idea of medicine "became the man, a Doctor of Medicine was Medicine itself" (p. 888). In short, Marsh must come to accept the inherent fallibility of other people and, more importantly, of himself. In doing so, he is able to begin to accept and know himself, not as a stranger but as a man, competent but limited and liable to failure.

The emotional coming-of-age that Marsh has been prepared for is fully achieved as he joins the townspeople who are searching for a missing hunter. Marsh becomes lost himself, so totally and frighteningly lost that he yearns for people, realizes that he needs them, and recognizes his kinship with others. Found by the other searchers, Marsh returns from the wilderness possessed of a new stability, a new appreciation of and growing love for his wife, a new understanding of himself and others.

With disarming predictability, Thompson ends the novel and completes Marsh's metamorphosis from doctor-as-instrument to a humane healer by introducing still another epidemic (this time meningitis), which unites all factions of the community in a battle against death. At the center of the battle is Lucas Marsh, no longer alone, no longer isolated and intolerant, no longer a stranger to himself or to others. The novel's final words, melodramatic as they are, prove an apt finale to the long, unwinding tale of the making of the quintessential, idealized doctor:

> The sick were waiting. The maimed and the dying, the stupid and the brilliant, the lucky and the blind...
> Ahead was the future.
> He picked up his bag and went out in the world and began the practice of Medicine. (p. 948)

Though frequently overburdened by Thompson's lack of restraint, *Not As A Stranger* is a prototypic example of the essential form of the medical novel. Similarly, Taylor Caldwell's 1968 best-seller *Testimony of Two Men* (fifth on that year's list) is a prototype of the successful, formulaic, and historically oriented medical idealization. Caldwell's novel, among the least artistically successful of its genre, is remarkable, not for memorable characterizations or for the successful creation of a fully realized fictional world, but rather for its reliance on and exploitation of the full range of formulaic elements handed down through the previous half-century by the various creators of fictionalized medical worlds. Reminiscent of *Dr. Nye of North Ostable* in its treatment of a good doctor who has been greviously wronged, *Testimony of Two Men* chronicles the fortunes of the misanthropic and ruthlessly honest Jonathan Ferrier, whose demands for perfection in both colleagues and friends are much like those of Lucas Marsh. Also like Marsh, Ferrier passes through a lengthy period of intense isolation, and after falling in love, he finds that his hatred is pierced and that he is able to reclaim his place within the community that has wronged him.[34]

Superimposed upon this basic and by 1968 familiar plot are melodramatic elements that Caldwell weaves into a ponderous historical tapestry. Among the most predictable of these are Ferrier's abuse at the hands of his vicious and bewitching wife, Mavis, whose death is rumored to have been his responsibility. Further entanglements arise from a subplot centered on Ferrier's hated brother, Harald, father of the child whose abortion killed Ferrier's unfaithful wife. Harald's guilt is a closely guarded secret, and its discovery by Ferrier leads the enraged doctor to attempt to murder his brother, an attempt stopped by Jenny Heger (p. 680), Haralds's stepdaughter and the young woman whom Ferrier comes to love and finally to marry.

Against the playing out of the romantic melodrama that is the core of the novel, Caldwell provides a predictable sequence of medical achievements and healing situations that establish the competence and altruistic goodness of the suffering and maligned Ferrier. Not only does he modernize the town's hospital (p. 123) and help the local medical community to police its own ranks, but he also saves both the life and soul of Francis Campion (p. 209), the suicidal son of Senator Campion, whose vendetta against Ferrier is aided by the influential Maurice Eaton, Mavis Ferrier's ostensible uncle who fears that he will be exposed as her real father (pp. 522–524).

Not content to paint her long-suffering hero as just a healer of body and soul, Caldwell also has him defend and aid the Irish poor (p. 295), tend to a friend who suffers from leprosy (pp. 273–281), revive and give the will to live to a grief-stricken professor (pp. 383–385), campaign against drug-addicted colleagues (p. 391), and finally, after being reconciled to the town that had wronged him, accept the post of chief surgeon at the local hospital (p. 699) and ultimately resume his practice (p. 702).

Having suffered so that he might learn self-awareness and compassion, Ferrier, whose furious detachment had sundered him from the human community, also learns to forgive and to love, and in learning these things, he is reborn and once again able to care for and help others. The novel, then, is a compendium of familiar devices and fictional types, and it succeeds, not because of its quality but because of the familiar paths it travels. Relying as had its generic predecessors on its intended audience's assumed desire to see yet again the life of a ruggedly individualistic and benevolent doctor, *Testimony of Two Men* demonstrates the inherent appeal of its central subject, an appeal that could even overcome the author's excesses and allow the story of Jonathan Ferrier to join the ranks of America's best-sellers.

7

Popular Culture: Proliferations

THE MULTIFORM IMAGE

Although it enjoyed a wide readership in the late 1960s, Taylor Caldwell's medical novel, *Testimony of Two Men,* became in 1977 a far more popular, far more widely known story, thanks to its transformation into a multiinstallment mini-series on network television and its subsequent reissue as a mass market paperback. Following the previous year's success of a number of serializations of lengthy novels, the television version of *Testimony* attracted millions of viewers who endured its convoluted plot and ponderous melodrama.

This dual transformation of Caldwell's medical world from a print into a nonprint and then back again into a print medium was not an unprecedented occurrence. Decades earlier, Max Brand's popular Dr. Kildare novels were translated into a number of successful movies and eventually into two different television series, first in the early 1960s and then again in the mid 1970s. Spurred by the popularity of the initial television series, Beagle Books reissued the seven Kildare novels in ninety-five-cent paperback editions. Also transformed into successful movies were Douglas's *Magnificent Obsession,* Thompson's *Not As A Stranger,* Green's *The Last Angry Man,* Richard Hooker's *M*A*S*H,* Frank G. Slaughter's *Doctor's Wives,* and Robin Cook's *Coma.*

The significance of such transformations, and of the many renderings of the idealized doctor image that followed, is that the more widely a dramatic image is presented to an increasingly large and diverse audience, the more likely that audience will be to respond to it. The response may come in gradual ways that in time allow people to assimilate and react to the shared experiences and implicit expectations presented. The impact and effect of such a wealth of portrayals are largely a result of what television critic Raymond Stedman calls a "cumulative factor." Although referring specifically to the popularity of television's daytime serials, Stedman's description is applicable to other formats in other media:

> The daytime serial, today as in the radio era, benefits from a cumulative factor. With each episode watched, the viewer invests more deeply in the undertaking. The continuing characters, expanded by the illusion of reality that accompanies the extended action, become as real as neighbors. More real, perhaps, because the viewer knows every secret . . . This detailed knowledge adds nuance to each piece of action, and it adds meaning that critics (who watch only occasionally, and clinically) cannot detect or appraise.[1]

This cumulative factor allows a mass audience, already familiar with similar vicarious experiences via previous exposures, to bring with it a wide range of emotional responses and expectations that are capitalized on by the media to provide a shared background against which new portrayals are presented.

In spite of the differences among the various media, the consistency and predictable sameness of the idealized image, as presented not only in the more traditional hardbound book but also in paperbacks, film, radio, and television, make possible an unprecedented amount of cultural sharing. That sharing, the result of media catering to an increasingly large and homogeneous audience, allows access to familiar constructs that are taken in and become a portion of people's everyday lives. The media provide an ever growing number of people with uncomplicated views of their complex worlds, views that in their simplistic and often distorted fashion hold much appeal and are accepted as part of the backdrop of day-to-day reality.[2] One of the most ubiquitous and readily available forms to present the idealized image of the American doctor during the past five decades has been the mass market paperback. Dating back to the Civil War, the inexpensive paperback novel has become a staple of American book publishing. After its initial success in the paperbound libraries of the late nineteenth century,[3] the paperback declined in popularity during the years between World War I (1914–18) and the end of the Great Depression in the 1930s. By 1939, however, Pocket Books "succeeded in bringing out paperbound editions of good books at 25 cents a copy."[4] The popularity of these cheap editions contributed to a paperback explosion that was fueled by a burst of wartime publishing, encouraged by the formation in 1942 of the Council on Books in Wartime, which worked to make books for the armed forces readily available.[5]

By the end of World War II (1945), the paperback was a familiar and increasingly popular part of the American reading public's diet, which often provided in quantity what it lacked in quality. Mass market paperbacks, like the best-sellers they often imitate, present detailed and particularized fictional worlds that are, in general, time-bound and become rapidly outdated. In fact, the success of the paperback novel in general, and particularly that of the medical idealization packaged in paperback format, is an illuminating example of the effects of technological possibilities and economic imperatives on the evolving form of an historically stable fictional type.

Just as the postwar economy came to rely more and more on the economic benefits derived from the interchangeability of assembly-line production and from planned obsolescence, so did the writers and publishers of mass market paperbacks come to realize that a growing reading public could be more easily persuaded to buy more and more books if those books were produced with careful attention to the interplay between apparent originality and underlying familiarity. Thus the capitalist-industrial model, which determined the production of more and more seemingly different varieties of the same basic products (whether automobiles or electric toothbrushes), also influenced the output of more and more mediocre novels that shared the same basic formula. They were presented in guises varied enough to appeal to a readership that wanted both the facade of diversity *and* the comfort of underlying sameness. Ironically, as it became more and more possible to diversify its product via new writers, new fictional techniques, and new interests in the reading public, the paperback industry found it desirable (because it was profitable) to base such diversity on what was already familiar and flourishing.

Astonishingly successful and enduring examples of the paperback industry's ability to capitalize on the continuous popularity of the stable and well-defined medical ideal are the novels of Elizabeth Seifert, Max Brand, and Frank G. Slaughter. Seifert and Slaughter, writing within a clearly defined formula that takes its major elements from the well-established idealization of the American doctor, have averaged more than one novel a year during the past four decades. Such an accomplishment attests not only to their energy but also to the enduring appeal of their genre. Max Brand, though far less prolific, made a lasting contribution to the genre with his dearly beloved physicians, Doctor Kildare and Doctor Gillespie.

Seifert is less popular than Slaughter in terms of total sales but is the more prolific of the two. She wrote more than eighty medical novels between 1938, when she published *Young Doctor Galahad* (winner of the $10,000 Dodd, Mead-Redbook prize), and 1982, when she completed *Two Doctors, Two Loves*. Even a partial list of her titles shows that they are less discrete entities than interchangeable parts of a larger and continuing fictional whole, a growing series that works and reworks familiar materials for an audience whose interests and tastes are relatively stable. The titles themselves are as predictable and repetitive as are the contents of the books, and what they offer to a reader is familiarity and the ease of knowing beforehand what will likely happen next. *Hillbilly Doctor, Army Doctor, Substitute Doctor,*

The New Doctor, Home-Town Doctor, and *Bachelor Doctor* provide the same easy fulfillment to reader expectations as do *Doctor Ellison's Decision, Doctor Woodward's Ambition, The Doctor's Bride, The Doctor's Confession, Doctor's Kingdom, Doctor's Destiny, The Doctor's Daughter, The Doctor's Affair*, and *The Doctor's Desperate Hour*, all of which recast the same basic characters in slightly altered plots and settings. Once familiar with the general outlines of a Seifert novel—an idealized doctor (usually young and almost always male) surmounts predictable obstacles and copes with familiar crises while strengthening his resolve and his ability to become the best possible healer at the same time that he triumphs in his tangled pursuit of true love—a reader who enjoys the formula can be sure of its repetition, whether the title is *Doctor of Mercy, Doctor at the Crossroads, A Doctor in the Family, A Doctor for Blue Jay Grove, Doctor on Trial*, or *Doctor With a Mission*. Having learned that the formula worked, Seifert did nothing to alter it, and her readers rewarded her with their loyalty.

A similar loyalty was tendered to Max Brand. During the years when Seifert was starting her career, he took time out from his successful pulp magazine stories to produce the seven Dr. Kildare novels that would make him famous as they underwent continual transformations through several of the mass media. Reputed to have written one-and-a-half million words per year during his thirty-year-career,[6] Brand gave little attention to the subtleties of characterization or careful plotting in the Kildare series. Instead, he took an already known and established fictional type, focused his attention on creating a bond of loyalty between the wise old Dr. Gillespie and the headstrong but talented young Dr. Kildare, and set in motion a series of episodic, sloppily plotted, evidently rushed, but remarkably popular medical novels.

As does Seifert, Brand relies heavily on his audience's familiarity with the conventions of the medical idealization, and by doing so he is able to save time, energy, and words. The shared familiarity allows Brand to begin his novels with an abruptness that catches and holds a reader's interest as it elicits a willing participation in the actual creation of the novel's ambiance. Typical of Brand's method is *The Secret of Dr. Kildare* which begins with characteristic abruptness: "The patients who came from the ends of the earth to consult Dr. Leonard Gillespie had been drawn to him by his fame as a miracle-worker or sent by baffled physicians of every country." Having established Gillespie's aura, Brand takes only one sentence to set up the novel's basic plot device—something is wrong with Gillespie and patients are being brought "not into the stormy presence of the great man, but to the young intern, James Kildare"—before going on to characterize the neophyte who is clearly destined to become a great and worthy successor to his mentor. The introductory description of Kildare also takes only one sentence: "He was neither very big nor very noisy and as a rule he failed to impress the people who had been drawn by a famous name; only a small minority saw in him that penetrating flash, that swiftly working instinct which seems almost foreknowledge and is characteristic of the born diagnostician".[7] Once Kildare is presented, the novel can get underway.

In less than half a page, Brand sketches in the broad outlines of his major characters, establishes the basic plot line, and foreshadows the resolution of the entire novel, all with a tempo that is clearly a holdover from his magazine writing and that would serve him well when he went on to write for Hollywood. That tempo characterizes all seven Kildare novels, each of which allows the reader to follow the good young doctor through a particular stage of his professional and personal growth. The evolution of Kildare binds the novels together into a coherent whole that is far more memorable than any of its component parts. Thus, in their original form, the novels—*Dr. Kildare's Trial, Young Dr. Kildare, Dr. Kildare Takes Charge, Calling Dr. Kildare, The Secret of Dr. Kildare, Dr. Kildare's Crisis,* and *Dr. Kildare's Search*—form a familiar series of interlocking parts. Their cumulative effect foreshadowed the even greater effectiveness that would eventually accrue when film and television adapted Brand's work to their own presentations.

Similar to the Kildare series in its relying on and benefitting from the cumulative effect of numerous interchangeable parts is the whole canon of medical novels by Frank G. Slaughter, who has been called America's "third most popular novelist." His total combined hardbound and paperback book sales (reputed to exceed 50,000,000 copies) place him, along with Earle Stanley Gardner and Erskine Caldwell, among the most successful (that is, most bought) of American writers.[8] Slaughter's success comes less from his ability to write well than from his knack for anticipating and then providing what his readers will buy. Like Brand, Slaughter, by his own admission, takes care to "keep the story moving" even at the expense of developing character or setting, and he works determinedly to make his medical worlds "intensely realistic."[9] Part of that realism, superficial though it is, comes from his own medical background (he retired from active practice in 1946), part of it from his attempt to avoid "writing the same story over and over again," which leads him to seek "out areas of history in which [he's] never worked before and in them lay new novels."[10]

Ironically, although Slaughter consistently fails in his attempt to avoid repeating the same basic story, he does manage to provide just enough superficial variety to keep his readers coming back. Relying as do both Seifert and Brand on the cumulative effect of the well-established conventions of the medical genre, Slaughter further capitalizes on his audience's liking for both exotic historicism and immediate contemporaneity by setting his novels in distant times and places as well as in the immediate present. The end result is a continuous stream of interchangeable doctors who share the same virtues, mouth the same platitudes, face the same problems, and offer the same solutions and comfort regardless of their given fictional world's locale or varied contours.

In his first novel, *That None Should Die* (1941), Slaughter created in young Dr. Ran Warren the prototypic idealization that he would recreate in novel after novel for the next forty years. Warren, a skilled and dedicated surgeon, plays out the role of rugged individualist in his fight against inept governmental control of the medical profession. In the course of his battle, like all of Slaughter's doctors to follow, Warren learns quickly from his mentors, fights various kinds of incompetence, places his patients' welfare before his own well-being, suffers from and resolves the complications in his love life, and emerges older, wiser, and altogether the miracle worker. In the final scene, familiar to followers of the genre, Warren is "in the operating theater again, gowned and masked, the blessed life-saving steel shining in his gloved hands. He was waiting for the anesthetist's nod, waiting to perform once more the miracle of surgery upon the figure beneath the sterile drapings. Working always toward the time when none should die for lack of the healing magic of the scalpel."[11]

The "healing magic" remains a constant throughout all of Slaughter's medical novels, and, considering his own surgical background, it is not surprising that the agent of that magic is often a skilled surgeon, sometimes torn by the conflict of the Civil War (Dr. Julian Chisholm of *In a Dark Garden*, 1946), or enmeshed in romantic entanglements during World War II (Captain Rick Winter, U.S. Army Medical Corps, in *Battle Surgeon*, 1944), or fighting a charge of treason during the Korean War (Captain Paul Scott in *Sword and Scalpel*, 1957). Also among Slaughter's gallery of surgeons is the title character of *Spencer Brade, M.D.* (1942), who must win the love of the woman whom he had originally married only for money before he can fully capitalize on his skill as the ideal surgeon, "a perfect machine, infused with humanity."[12] Kindred souls to Brade in that their dedication and magical skill are temporarily diverted from their true course by romantic entanglements that are eventually resolved are Dr. Dan Carter (*The Healer*, 1955), Dr. Mike Constant (*A Savage Place*, 1964), and Dr. Bruce Graham (*Surgeon, U.S.A.*, 1966), all of whom are basically the same character, putting on different names and different costumes while enacting the same basic adventures.

Slaughter may place his young doctors in the midst of the Spanish Inquisition (*Divine Mistress*, 1949) or pull them into the arena of contemporary medical and social problems—medical politics in *Convention M.D.* (1972), the decay of a greatly needed urban hospital in *Code Five* (1971), the controversy over the patient's right to die in *Women in White* (1974), or the battle between medical science and a potentially catastrophic outbreak of an ancient disease in *Plague Ship* (1976). But in all of these, and despite their superficial variety, the basic drama of the skilled, dedicated, and idealized doctor is played out within the same framework that had been evolving since the years when Oliver Wendell Holmes and S. Weir Mitchell first presented the American reading public with their doctors of good character.

Still more varied examples of superficially diverse portrayals of the stable ideal can be found in the raft of medical paperbacks that appear routinely on mass market racks in grocery, drug, stationery, and department stores, bus and train station newsstands, and airport gift shops. The paperback medical novel often must compete for attention with slick magazines and other paperbacks that cater to readers' tastes for sex, violence, and the bizarre. As a result, the present-day descendants of such doctors as Kittredge, North, and Leslie are slickly packaged between glossy covers that often promise more titillation than they deliver.

What the paperbacks do deliver are variations on the theme of the good doctor triumphing over nearly insurmountable odds to save patients, aid the community, rehabilitate other talented but fallen doctors, pioneer in medical breakthroughs, and perform the all-but-miraculous procedure that once again elevates him to godlike heights. Anxious to please their restless audiences, the authors concentrate on keeping their doctors' exploits timely and provocative. The result, as already noted, is novels with interchangeable plots and characters, the sum total of which is, as with the novels of Seifert and Slaughter, far more memorable than any of its several parts.

There are the romantic melodramas (*Doctors and Wives, Resort M.D., Cruise Ship M.D., The Doctor Who Made House Calls*)[13] in which the good doctor's career is jeopardized by a love affair that must be set right before he can again function effectively. Also concerned with careers in jeopardy are novels about malpractice (*The Clinic, Malpractice, A Wilderness of Monkeys*) and peer review (*The Death Committee*);[14] in these, the good doctor is invariably vindicated after enduring and triumphing over assorted though predictable hardships. Another form of medical triumph occurs in novels whose plots center around either experimental medicine (*The Clewiston Test, The Experiment, The Terminal Man*) or the ethical questions posed by prolonging life with extraordinary measures (*Ward 402*).[15] Less exotic but still providing a backdrop for idealization are novels that chronicle the decay and rejuvenation of a vital city hospital (*The Hospital Makers*), show the frustrations and joys of practicing in a rural clinic (*Four Doctors*), and present the difficulties and the elation of medical training (*The Interns, Intern*).[16]

Moving away, though only ostensibly, from more familiar patterns in order, finally, to reassert the viability of the underlying ideal are those medical novels that enliven their tales with a renewed trace of the diabolical. In them, misguided science and the malevolent doctor threaten catastrophic harm until all is made right by a modernized version of the doctor of skill, concern, and good character. The master of this subgenre is Robin Cook, himself a physician, who has gauged well his readers' unfailing appetite for a mix of timely malevolence, the bizarre, and the familiarly benign. In *Coma* (1977), Cook's first and prototypic medical thriller, the idealized doctor is transformed into a young woman medical student of dedication, clear sight, and courage. She uncovers a Rappaccini-like plot to induce coma in patients whose bodies are then "harvested" for organs needed for transplant research. Risking her life and fighting a malign medical establishment, she hurtles through outlandishly suspenseful adventures as she works to crush the medical menace she has discovered.

For all its updated and high-tech trappings, *Coma* and its benevolent and dedicated doctor-in-training remain as modernized variants of familiar types and themes. The malevolence of Hawthorne's Unpardonable Sinners resurfaces in Cook's novel and is, after much heat and light, extinguished by the familiar doctor of good character and determination. With a keen eye to his reading public, Cook elaborated on the formula established in *Coma* and turned out a stream of medical thrillers—*Brain* (1981), *Fever* (1982), *Godplayer* (1983), *Mindbend* (1985)—all presenting the familiar idealization pitted against contemporary but fallible malevolence.

Other writers were quick to try to capitalize on the popularity of Cook's novels. Those with less skill but more grotesque imaginations devised medical worlds that encompass (say the cover blurbs) "the world's best kept medical secret...[and] the most deadly" (*Side Effects*, 1985); a plot of "excrutiating medical horror" involving illicit brain transplants (*The Donors*, 1982); a neurophysiologist's "obscene procedure" that is "the most shocking medical experiment of all time (*Heads*, 1985); and an expose of fetal transplants, cloning, and the exploitation and destruction of surrogate mothers (*The Cradle Will Fall*, 1980).[17]

For all of the blood, gore, and horror that fill these literary copycats, the fundamental image of the good doctor remains central. Over and over in book after book, the third-and even fourth-generation descendents of those benevolent, talented, and godly doctors—whatever their contemporary guise— continue to practice their art and to appeal to a large and loyal audience that finds them often more attractive, more compassionate, and more desirable than it finds its doctors in real life.

8

Popular Culture: Familiar Differences

TELEVISION DOCTORS: THE ULTIMATE FORM

As extensive as it is, the popularity of America's paperback doctors and their fictional ancestors is overshadowed by the visibility of the idealized physicians who inhabit the medical worlds of network television. Because of its ability to reach a mass audience, television has been able to present its doctors to far more people than were ever exposed to similar characterizations in any other medium. Furthermore, because of its unique characteristics, television has shown the apotheosis of the doctor in forms more potent and potentially more persuasive than any ever before created.

Part of television's impact comes from the growth of its mass audience. In 1950, about one hundred television stations were broadcasting programs to nearly 5,000,000 television sets. In 1956, 450 stations were serving 37,000,000 sets. By 1963, there were more than 600 stations and 56,000,000 sets, and in 1970, 850 stations were received by over 84,000,000 sets. By 1986, 904 commercial and 209 educational stations were broadcasting to 87,590,000 sets. By then, 98 percent of American homes had at least one set. The average daily viewing time in 1975 exceeded six hours and increased to over seven hours by 1985. Weekly viewing time in 1985 for all people averaged 31 hours and 28 minutes. Year by year, as this steady increase continued, so did the overall effect of electronic influence. As Giraud Chester has pointed out,

Now virtually all American homes are equipped with at least one television set; more than one-quarter of these households has two or more sets. In the average home, people watch television almost six hours a day. From morning through the late evening hours, television now commands the "strongest sustained attention" of most American families.[1]

Both the size of the audience *and* its seemingly insatiable viewing habits lead to an unprecedented amount of cultural sharing: "Never before have such large and varied publics ... shared so much of the same cultural system of messages and images, and the assumptions embedded in them. Television offers a universal curriculum that everyone can learn."[2] The content of that "universal curriculum," intensified by the form of its presentation, has made television a social force of enormous magnitude precisely because it has become an integral part of so many people's everyday lives. What viewers experience in their everyday television watching is often considerably different from what they experience in real life. According to critic Harry M. Brown, television's view of life is unreal in three particular ways: the medium "prolongs youth and youthful values"; it "promotes idealism"; and it "shows how the impossible can be achieved, not once but time and time again as a matter of routine."[3]

The routine achievement of the impossible and the near-impossible has been a hallmark of television's doctors, and the distortions evident in their medical worlds are similar to the kinds of distortions that have characterized the medium's portrayal of other groups of workers. In 1964 Melvin DeFleur studied the world of work as presented on television and determined that "as a learning source ... television content that deals with occupational roles can be characterized as selective, unreal, stereotyped, and misleading."[4] Little if anything has changed since then to right these media wrongs. Such distortions, routinely presented to a receptive mass audience, have great potential for affecting people's attitudes and expectations about the everyday world around them. Because it is increasingly able "to dominate [the nation's] symbol producing apparatus," television is more and more able "to create the ambience that forms consciousness itself."[5] With such power American television, especially from the late 1960s through the mid–1980s, nurtured the final flowering of the idealized doctor in presentations that simultaneously shared and further exaggerated the image that had been evolving for a full century.

Television's most popular doctors have appeared in several varieties, yet they share the same core of ideal and familiar characteristics. Seen far more often than the average viewer's own physician, these electronic doctors work in a world of medical care for surpassing anything in real life. They usually save lives with ease, mend marriages, reconcile alienated families, give patients the will to live, and continuously reassert the primacy of the doctor-patient relationship. As drama, the medical shows fall far short of greatness, but as delineations of an ideal, they cannot be faulted. Although there are occasional snatches of dialogue that hint at a lesser reality, more typical are the continual allusions to the doctor's divinity: " 'A patient will reach for God, or His more earthbound and vulnerable substitute, the doctor' "; " 'The trouble with doctors is that patients turn us into Gods before we become men' "; " 'It's a sacred gift you have, doctor' "; " 'He's not dead until I say he's dead.' "[6]

Patients live more often than not (they die only from incurable disease); doctors rarely if ever fail, and if they begin to err, they are presented as atypical and quickly brought back into the fold by their more level-headed and representative colleagues; the medical system seldom falters in its task of bringing the best possible care to all people. In short, the world of the television doctor is a medical utopia unmatched in previous idealization or in real life.

Whether to the research institute of "The Doctors" segment of "The Bold Ones," or to the university medical complex of "Medical Center," or to the spacious and soothing offices of "Marcus Welby, M.D.," patients come in pain and distress and go, by show's end, in good health and high spirits. The cast of characters, the disease, and the mode of treatment may change from week to week and from show to show, but the overall pattern of care and medical idealization remains as unchanging as it does in the novels of Slaughter and Seifert and in the medical best-sellers.

Television's own "best-seller" was "Marcus Welby, M.D.," whose continuing popularity during its prime-time years on the air (1969–76) was a result of the then-right combination of formulaic elements. Welby (perhaps too obviously well-named) had, as a general practitioner, a closer and more complete relationship with his patients than did the surgeons and other specialists of "Medical Center" and "The Bold Ones." Also, the locales of these latter shows—a university medical center and a private research institute—though they were more contemporary and let the shows incorporate the latest advances in medical technology, were less familiar and potentially more stressful to viewers than was the home-based office of Dr. Welby.

In its choice of Robert Young to play Welby, ABC made its smartest decision about the series. Young brought to the role not only the proper look of age and calm expertise, but also the aura of patient wisdom and fairness that his audience associated with his earlier portrayal of Jim Anderson in the radio and television series, "Father Knows Best." Neither of the other major medical shows was able to capitalize nearly so well on the talents of its senior colleagues: "Medical Center's" Dr. Paul Lochner (James Daly) was primarily an administrator and his role was clearly secondary; Dr. David Craig (E. G. Marshall) of "The Bold Ones" shared the spotlight with two younger colleagues. Only Young/Welby was able to capitalize on his age.

Because he was older, wiser, calmer, more benevolent, and often priestlike, Welby was able to teach and counsel his younger colleague, Dr. Steven Kiley (played by James Brolin). In this relationship as in those with his patients, Welby was the one who knew best, and both Kiley and the patients benefitted. The extent to which Young's characterization of Welby struck a responsive chord among viewers and among the medical profession was evident in the show's top-ranked Nielsen ratings and in the special awards that it received from the American Medical Association and the American Academy of Family Physicians. Another indication of its effect was the fact that 250,000 letters, most of them requesting medical advice, were sent by viewers to "Dr. Marcus Welby" during the first five years of his TV practice.[7]

Further enhancing "Welby's" popularity was the show's ability to present viewers with superficial change and variety within a larger framework of sameness and familiarity. In the early years, one of Welby's chief tasks was to professionalize fully the motorcycle-riding Dr. Kiley, who lacked patience and good judgment and who often disagreed with but invariably came to defer to the older and wiser Welby. This "education of the neophyte" subplot gave viewers a double reward: it presented Welby at his wisest and most benevolent, and it showed Kiley maturing and becoming more and more the ideal type epitomized by his mentor.

The maturing of young Dr. Kiley led to another superficial change in the show at the beginning of the 1974–75 season when Welby took on the added role of advisor to a family practice clinic. This new facet of his career allowed him to offer sage advice to intense but untried residents, something he could no longer do with Kiley, who had by then profited from Welby's counsel, had given up his motorcycle, and had become thoroughly professionalized and conservative.

Yet even with these changes, the show remained essentially what it had always been—a tour de force for Welby and for the idealization he represented. In the first show of that 1974–75 season, Welby found it necessary to say to a second-year resident disturbed by an intransigent patient, "We're only human," a statement reserved for situations where Welby's medicine and ideal manner fail (but only temporarily) to resolve a given week's dilemma. By show's end, the patient had been pacified and was willing to accept treatment, the resident had learned the need to view his patients as complex entities, and Welby had proven that he (and by extension his profession) could yet again do all.

It was the repeated and demonstrated ability to do all, week after week, year after year, that made Welby and other television doctors—Kiley, Gannon, Lochner, Craig, Stuart, Hunter, and others—such potent manifestations of the ideal doctor. In their bloodless and usually deathless medical worlds, all that a real-life patient could hope for occurred with regularity. The cumulative effect of these idealizations went far to reinforce the beliefs of viewers, who slowly but assuredly came to admire, eventually to hope for, and finally to expect what could be found only in the soothing and ideal medical worlds of Marcus Welby and his video colleagues.

CONCLUDING VIEWS: CONTINUITY AND CHANGE

After the spring of 1976 when both "Marcus Welby, M.D." and "Medical Center" were dropped from their prime-time slots ("The Doctors" segment of "The Bold Ones" had been cancelled at the end of the 1972–73 season), television viewers were treated to a varied assortment of medical worlds, none proving entirely satisfactory, all with little success and short runs. NBC launched "Medical Story" in response to the short success of its documentary-styled "Police Story," but found that excessive realism and a changing cast of doctors did nothing but insure that the show would leave the air midway through its first season. Attempts at situation comedy grafted onto a medical setting—starring Danny Thomas as an eccentric G.P. and Brian Keith as a pediatrician in Hawaii—were quick to leave the screen, as was the appearance of James Franciscus as a doctor in a western setting.

Trying to fill the void left by the removal of "Welby," ABC launched "Westside Medical" in the spring of 1977, touting it as a "new kind of medical drama." The network fragmented the show's focus by presenting three young doctors, none with enough experience or character to inspire trust or convey a lasting impression. The trio did not return for a second season. Similarly unsuccessful was "Rafferty" (CBS), whose title character, Dr. Sidney Rafferty, was an eccentric, blunt, and demanding surgeon who also maintained a private family practice with a young associate. The potential advantage of mixing the drama of a large hospital with the more pedestrian concerns of general practice was unable to counteract the sour character of Rafferty, and the show did not survive its first season in the fall of 1977.

The only medical show that did survive beyond its second season was "Quincy", but since its title character was a forensic pathologist, the show focused more on detective and police work than on anything akin to patient care. Another atypical variant was "A.E.S. Hudson Street," a situation comedy set in the emergency room of a large city hospital; it relied for its short-lived humor on the kind of mayhem generated by such crises as a hospitalwide power failure. Less dependent on sight gags and slapstick was "Julie Farr, M.D.," a spinoff from a moderately successful made-for-television movie called *Having Babies*. Though benefitting from its audience's interest in childbirth and infants, the show demonstrated that the combination of a woman doctor and a highly restricted medical specialty proved to be a liability in terms of long-term audience response. Julie Farr did not become another Marcus Welby.

The failure of these new and atypical medical shows to capture a large audience and gain its loyalty could have been predicted. None was able to survive the damage done by its deviation from the long-established and expected medical idealization. That idealization, having evolved for over a century, was deeply embedded in the public mind, and "since there is need to attract and hold an audience, the media cannot vary too much from the audience's expectations or values or desires."[8] In the case of these particular shows, too much variety of the wrong kinds came quickly to be the kiss of network death.

Realizing and taking heed of that singular fact, NBC was at last able in the 1982–83 season to launch "St. Elsewhere," nickname of the aging urban hospital that was the stage for the show's mixture of familiarity, novelty, and atypical quality. The audience's response was slow to gain momentum, and the network asserted that it was risking a second-season renewal in response to loyal but limited viewer pressure and also as part of its alleged dedication to "quality programming." By the end of the second season, the network's gamble paid off: "St. Elsewhere" was a money-making success, a popular hit that carried with it the added virtue of validating NBC's commitment to "quality."

What the show really exemplifed and what accounted for its "hit" status more than its quality or its occasional quirkiness was the continuing vitality and tenacious hold of the well-established tradition of medical idealization. For all of its new "realism" and superficially unusual characterizations, "St. Elsewhere" was wisely designed to portray its several doctors, for all their eccentricities, in basically the same heroic and idealized mode that had been handed down for generations. Even when it was being acerbic and iconoclastic, the show both relied on and extended the idealization rather than question it or establish a genuinely alternative view.

Composed as it was of the right elements, "St. Elsewhere" was rewarded by the viewing public, which granted the response that NBC had envisioned. That response, widespread and highly positive, arose from preexisting attitudes toward shared cultural forms. "St. Elsewhere's" medical world gave its viewers access to an ever-present past that continued to assert its attraction in a world changing at ever-increasing speed. Faced with such change and unwilling or unable to cope with all of it, people opted for an only superficially modernized version of a remembered and imagined past, accessible, at least from time to time, via this newly favored artifact. In "St. Elsewhere", viewers found a new resting place, an interesting spot that could satisfy both their curiosity for something new and their more deeply engrained longing for the safe and familiar.

Thus, as did its electronic predecessors and as will its inevitable descendents,[9] "St. Elsewhere" gives people at least vicarious access to an ideal medical world receding further and further from the realities of America's complex health care system. The actualities of that system, its strengths and its weaknesses, and the demands placed on it make the widespread desire for a television-like medical world less and less realistic, though understandable. Not only are such desires unrealistic, they are potentially detrimental to all concerned, since they are based on an outmoded world view that began as an idealization and has over the years been less and less in touch with reality.

The growing disparity between the hoped-for and the real creates problems in all areas of everyday life, not just in people's dealings with their doctors. That people prefer their dream worlds to a lesser reality is not surprising, especially when those dream worlds seem more able to fulfill the most basic and crucial human needs. What is troublesome, and in need of rethinking, is that people also allow their dream worlds to undermine the quality of real life and weaken their resolve and ability to effect needed and possible change. What is fondly remembered—from the real or vicarious past—needs to be seen for what it actually was. Then it needs to be set aside and replaced with a view of life that is closer to reality's contours.

In the particular case of the evolving image of the American doctor, neither the malevolent Rappaccini nor the benevolent and thoroughly idealized Dr. Kildare should be remembered for anything more than the cultural form each has become. To fear the evil of an Ethan Brand (or of his modern-day avatar, Dr. Harold Stark, in *Coma*) is as naive and counterproductive for a patient and his or her doctor as it is to hope for or imagine being a Dr. Kittredge or a Marcus Welby. Neither extreme has its place in people's everyday lives. Reality is a far preferable, and needed, alternative.

Notes

CHAPTER 1

1. John C. Burnham, "American Medicine's Golden Age: What Happened to It?" *Science*, 215 (March 19, 1982), 1474–79.

CHAPTER 2

1. Morris L. Cogan, "Toward A Definition of Profession," *Harvard Educational Review*, 23, No. 1 (Winter 1953), 33–50.

2. Geoffrey Millerson, *The Qualifying Associations: A Study in Professionalization* (New York: The Humanities Press, 1964), p. 13.

3. Millerson, p. 10.

4. Everett C. Hughes, "Professions," *Daedalus*, 92, No. 4 (Fall 1963), 656. More recent and less benign views of the nature and development of professions are evident in Gerald L. Geison, ed. *Professions and Professional Ideologies in America* (Chapel Hill: Univ. of North Carolina Press, 1983).

5. A. M. Carr-Saunders and P. A. Wilson, *The Professions* (Oxford: The Clarendon Press, 1933), p. 491.

6. Bernard Barber, "Some Problems in the Sociology of the Professions," *Daedalus*, 92, No. 4 (Fall 1963), 671.

7. Barber, p. 672.

8. Barber, p. 673. See Eliot Freidson, *Profession of Medicine: A Study of the Sociology of Applied Knowledge* (New York: Harper & Row, 1970), pp. 71–84 for a discussion of the formal characteristics of a profession and the sources of professional status.

9. Roy Lubove's *The Professional Altruist: The Emergence of Social Work as a Career 1880–1930* (New York: Atheneum Press, 1969) analyzes the evolution of social work from a voluntary philanthropic effort to a fully established profession and demonstrates that the process was completed only after American society became willing to accept and respond positively to social workers' own claims for profes-

sional status. Also see Burton J. Bledstein, *The Culture of Professionalism: The Middle Class and the Development of Higher Education in America* (New York: W. W. Norton, 1976), pp. 92–105 for a cogent description of the conservative effects of a profession's gaining esteem and influence.

10. Daniel H. Calhoun, *Professional Lives in America* (Cambridge, Mass: Harvard Univ. Press, 1965), p. 7.

11. Calhoun, p. 178.

12. Calhoun, p. 7.

13. Barber, p. 672.

14. This description of the characteristics of professions relies heavily on Millerson's *The Qualifying Associations: A Study in Professionalization*. That Millerson bases his discussion on the professions in England serves to emphasize that professions, in general and cross-culturally, share similar characteristics.

15. Millerson, pp. 29–31.

16. Millerson, p. 10. For a contrasting view of the efficacy of professional organizations, see Joseph F. Kett, *The Formation of the American Medical Profession: The Role of Institutions, 1780–1860* (New Haven: Yale Univ. Press, 1968).

17. See Howard S. Becker et al., eds., *Boys In White: Student Culture in Medical School* (Chicago: Univ. of Chicago Press, 1961), pp. 7ff.

18. Barber, pp. 674–75.

19. Robert K. Merton et al., eds., *The Student Physician: Introductory Studies in the Sociology of Medical Education* (Cambridge, Mass.: Harvard Univ. Press, 1957), p. vii.

20. Elton Rayack, *Professional Power and American Medicine: The Economics of the American Medical Association* (New York: World Publ. Co., 1967), p. xiv.

21. Oliver Garceau, *The Political Life of the American Medical Association* (Hamden, Conn.: Archon Books, 1961), p. 167. Perceptive and thought-provoking views of the past quarter-century's increased skepticism of and disenchantment with the professions are available in Thomas L. Haskell, ed. *The Authority of Experts: Studies in History and Theory* (Bloomington: Univ. of Indiana Press, 1984).

22. Samuel W. Bloom, "Some Implications of Studies in the Professionalization of the Physician," in E. Gartly Jaco, ed., *Patients, Physicians, and Illness* (New York: The Free Press, 1958), p. 313.

23. Arthur K. Davis, "Bureaucratic Patterns in the Navy Officer Corps," *Social Forces*, 27 (Dec. 1948), 143–53, quoted in Bloom, "Some Implications . . . ," p. 313.

24. Becker et al., p. 94.

25. Becker et al., p. 111.

26. Becker et al., p. 134.

27. Becker et al., p. 163.

28. Patricia L. Kendall and H. C. Selvin, "Tendencies Toward Specialization in Medical Training," in Merton et al., pp. 155–62.

29. Kendall and Selvin, p. 174. Also see Paul Starr, *The Social Transformation of American Medicine* (New York: Basic Books, Inc., 1982), pp. 355–359 for an elaboration of structural factors within the medical profession that contributed to the increase in specialization.

30. Renee C. Fox, "Training for Uncertainty," in Merton, et al., p. 208.

31. Fox, p. 216.

32. Becker et al., pp. 223–27, 234.

33. Mary Jean Huntington, "The Development of a Professional Self-Image," in Merton et al., p. 181.

34. Huntington, p. 183.

35. Peter L. Berger and Thomas Luckmann, *The Social Construction of Reality* (Garden City, N.Y.: Anchor Books, 1967), p. 132.

36. William Martin, "Preferences for Types of Patients," in Merton et al., p. 204.

37. See Samuel W. Bloom, *The Doctor and His Patient* (New York: The Free Press, 1965) for a thorough discussion of the doctor-patient relationship as a system of culturally derived social roles. Although Bloom provides a useful schema for analyzing the multiple forces affecting doctors and patients, he deemphasizes the importance of those elements of the relationship that remain essentially static in face of the other variables within the relationship. Also see Eliot Freidson, *Professional Dominance: The Social Structure of Medical Care* (New York: Aldine Publ. Co., 1970); Freidson argues persuasively that the structural characteristics of the profession, i.e., its organization, are more influential than either goodwill or skill in determining the quality and availability of medical care.

38. Henry D. Lederer, "How the Sick View Their World," in Jaco, pp. 249–50.

39. Becker et al., p. 238.

40. Carr-Saunders and Wilson, p. 104.

41. Talcott Parsons, *The Social System* (Glencoe, Ill.: The Free Press, 1951), p. 446.

42. Parsons, p. 435.

43. See Eliot Freidson, *Patients' Views of Medical Practice* (Chicago: Univ. of Chicago Press, 1980). Freidson's entire ninth chapter (Dilemmas in the Doctor-Patient Relationship) presents a clear view of how changes in the field of medicine have tended to erode that crucial relationship. Also see Kenneth Ludmerer's *Learning to Heal* (New York: Basic Books, Inc., 1985) for a fuller view of the changes and continuities in American medical education.

CHAPTER 3

1. Useful bibliographical essays on American medical history appear in Erwin H. Ackernecht, M.D., *A Short History of Medicine*, rev. ed. (New York: The Ronald Press, 1968) and in Charles E. Rosenberg, *The Cholera Years: America in 1832, 1849, 1866* (Chicago: Univ. of Chicago Press, 1962). Further background on the social dimensions of American medical practice is available in Rosemary Stevens, *American Medicine and the Public Interest* (New Haven: Yale Univ. Press, 1971); John Duffy, *The Healers: The Rise of the Medical Establishment* (New York: McGraw-Hill, 1976); Morris J. Vogel and Charles E. Rosenberg, eds., *The Therapeutic Revolution: Essays in the Social History of American Medicine* (Philadelphia: Univ. of Pennsylvania Press, 1979); Paul Starr, *The Social Transformation of American Medicine* (New York: Basic Books, Inc., 1982); and Judith Walzer Leavitt and Ronald L. Numbers, eds., *Sickness and Health in America*, 2nd. ed., rev. (Madison: Univ. of Wisconsin Press, 1985). Also of good use are Kenneth Ludmerer, *Learning to Heal* (New York: Basic Books, Inc., 1985); Regina Markell Morantz-Sanchez, *Sympathy and Science: Women Physicians in American Medicine* (New York: Oxford Univ. Press, 1987); and Edward Shorter, *Bedside Manners: The Troubled History of Doctors and Patients* (New York: Simon and Schuster, 1987).

2. Richard Harrison Shryock, "The Medical History of the American People,"

in *Medicine in America: Historical Essays* (Baltimore: Johns Hopkins Press, 1961), p. 5.

3. Shryock, "The Medical History of the American People," p. 4.

4. Richard Harrison Shryock, *Medicine and Society in America 1660–1860* (New York: New York Univ. Press, 1960), p. 10.

5. Shryock, *Medicine and Society*, p. 15.

6. Shryock, *Medicine and Society*, p. 9.

7. Shryock, *Medicine and Society*, p. 8.

8. Shryock, *Medicine and Society*, p. 44.

9. Shryock, *Medicine and Society*, p. 47.

10. Shryock, "The Medical History of the American People," p. 8.

11. Shryock, *Medicine and Society*; see pp. 18–58 for a general discussion of the medical situation in the colonial period.

12. Richard Harrison Shryock, *The Development of Modern Medicine* (New York: Alfred A. Knopf, 1947), p. 69. Also see Martin Kaufman, *American Medical Education: The Formative Years, 1765–1910* (Westport, Conn.: Greenwood Press, 1976); William Frederick Norwood, *Medical Education in the United States Before the Civil War* (Philadelphia: Univ. of Pennsylvania Press, 1944); and Morris J. Vogel and Charles E. Rosenberg, eds., *The Therapeutic Revolution: Essays in the Social History of American Medicine* (Philadelphia: Univ. of Pennsylvania Press, 1979).

13. Shryock, *Medicine and Society*, p. 20.

14. Shryock, *Medicine and Society*, p. 31.

15. Shryock, *Medicine and Society*, p. 38.

16. Charles E. Rosenberg, *The Cholera Years: America in 1832, 1849, 1866* (Chicago: Univ. of Chicago Press, 1962), pp. 70–71. Also see John Harley Warner, *The Therapeutic Perspective: Medical Practice, Knowledge, and Professional Identity in America, 1820–1865* (Cambridge, Mass.: Harvard Univ. Press, 1986).

17. Shryock, *Medicine and Society*, p. 104.

18. Rosenberg (p. 40) demonstrates persuasively that Americans had to free themselves from the belief that disease was a natural result of a sinful life before preventive medicine could be recognized as a necessary adjunct of health care. Not until disease was viewed as something other than an exercise of God's will were public health measures able to gain appreciable support.

19. Rosenberg, p. 65.

20. Rosenberg, p. 68.

21. Rosenberg, p. 222.

22. Henry E. Sigerist, *American Medicine* (New York: W. W. Norton, 1934), p. 133.

23. Richard Harrison Shryock, "The American Physician in 1846 and 1946: A Study in Professional Contrasts," in *Medicine in America*, p. 154. Also see Duffy.

24. Shryock, *The Development of Modern Medicine*, p. 258.

25. Joseph F. Kett, *The Formation of the American Medical Profession: The Role of Institutions, 1780–1860* (New Haven: Yale Univ. Press, 1968), pp. 170–71.

26. Shryock, "The American Physician in 1846 and 1946," p. 157. Also see Duffy.

27. Shryock, *The Development of Modern Medicine*, pp. 250–55.

28. Shryock, *Medicine and Society*, pp. 143–48.

29. Shryock, *The Development of Modern Medicine*, p. 248.

30. Shryock, "The American Physician in 1846 and 1946," p. 171.

31. Kett, p. 167.

32. Daniel H. Calhoun, *Professional Lives in America: Structure and Aspiration 1750–1850* (Cambridge, Mass.: Harvard Univ. Press, 1965), p. 21.

33. Kett, p. 170.

34. Kett, pp. 176–77.

35. Kett, p. 171.

36. Kett, p. 172.

37. Richard Harrison Shryock, "The Interplay of Social and Internal Factors in Modern Medicine: An Historical Analysis," in *Medicine in America: Historical Essays*, pp. 313ff.

38. Ackerknecht, p. 225.

39. Shryock, "The Medical History of the American People," pp. 22ff.

40. Ronald L. Numbers, "The Fall and Rise of the American Medical Profession," in Leavitt and Numbers, p. 189. Also see Robert P. Hudson, "Abraham Flexner in Perspective: American Medical Education, 1865–1910" in Leavitt and Numbers, pp. 148–58 and Kenneth Ludmerer, *Learning to Heal* (New York: Basic Books, Inc., 1985).

41. Shryock, *The Development of Modern Medicine*, p. 314.

42. Shryock, *The Development of Modern Medicine*, p. 318.

43. Shryock, *The Development of Modern Medicine*, pp. 338, 351. Also see John C. Burnham, "American Medicine's Golden Age: What Happened to It?" *Science*, 215 (March 19, 1982), 1474–79.

44. Robert H. Wiebe, *The Search for Order 1877–1920* (New York: Hill and Wang, 1969), passim. In addition to Wiebe's fine study, useful introductions to the period in which the American nation became a bureaucratized system of continuity, regularity, functionality, and rationality can be found in Gabriel Kolko's *The Triumph of Conservatism* (Chicago: Quadrangle Books, 1967); Roy Lubove's *The Professional Altruist* (New York: Atheneum, 1969); James Weinstein's *The Corporate Ideal in the Liberal State: 1900–1918* (Boston: Beacon Press, 1969), William Appleman Williams' *The Contours of American History* (Chicago: Univ. of Chicago Press, 1966), and Burton J. Bledstein, *The Culture of Professionalism: The Middle Class and the Development of Higher Education in America* (New York: W. W. Norton, 1976).

45. Wiebe, p. 115.

46. Shryock, "The Medical History of the American People," p. 31. Also see Robert P. Hudson, "Abraham Flexner in Perspective: American Medical Education, 1865–1910," in Leavitt and Numbers, pp. 148–158.

47. James Weinstein, *The Corporate Ideal in the Liberal State: 1900–1918* (Boston: Beacon Press, 1969), p. 61.

48. Weinstein, pp. 33, 137–38. Also see Paul Starr, *The Social Transformation of American Medicine* (New York: Basic Books, Inc., 1982), Book One, Chapter Six, "Escape From the Corporation, 1900–1930."

49. Wayne G. Menke, "The Doctor: Change and Conflict in American Medical Practice," diss., University of Minnesota, 1961, pp. xiv et passim.

50. Shryock, "The Development of Modern Medicine," p. 419.

51. Everett C. Hughes, "Professions," *Daedalus*, 92, No. 4 (Fall 1963), 655.

52. Menke, p. 328.

53. Shryock, *The Development of Modern Medicine*, p. 384.

54. Edmund K. Faltermayer, "Better Care at Less Cost Without Miracles," *Fortune*, LXXXI, No. 1 (Jan. 1970), 80.

55. Dan Cordtz, "Change Begins in the Doctor's Office," *Fortune*, LXXXI, No. 1 (Jan. 1970), 85–86.

56. Paul Starr, *The Social Transformation of American Medicine* (New York: Basic Books, Inc. 1982), pp. 420–25.

57. Godfrey Hodgson, "The Politics of American Health Care," *The Atlantic*, 232, No. 4 (October 1973), p. 56.

58. Typical of the genre are Richard Carter, *The Doctor Business* (New York: Doubleday, 1958); Fred J. Cook, *The Plot Against the Patient* (Englewood Cliffs, N.J.: Prentice-Hall, Inc., 1967); Barbara Ehrenreich and John Ehrenreich, *The American Health Empire: Power, Profits and Politics* (New York: Random House, 1970); Senator Edward M. Kennedy, *In Critical Condition* (New York: Pocket Books, 1973); William Michelfelder, *It's Cheaper to Die* (New York: George Braziller, 1960); Roul Tunley, *The American Health Scandal* (New York: Harper & Row, 1966); and James Harvey Young, *The Medical Messiahs: A Social History of Health Quackery in Twentieth-Century America* (Princeton, N.J.: Princeton Univ. Press, 1967). Characteristic of earlier and more strident critiques are E. M. Josephson, *Your Life is Their Toy*, 2nd. ed. (New York: Chedney Press, 1948); John L. Spivak, *The Medical Trust Unmasked* (New York: Louis S. Siegfried, 1929); and Henry R. Strong, *The Machinations of the American Medical Association* (St. Louis: The National Druggist, 1909).

59. Shryock, *The Development of Modern Medicine*, p. 431.

60. Eli Ginzberg with Miriam Ostow, *Men, Money, and Medicine* (New York: Columbia Univ. Press, 1969), p. 85. Also see Morris J. Vogel and Charles E. Rosenberg, eds., *The Therapeutic Revolution: Essays in the Social History of American Medicine* (Philadelphia: Univ. of Pennsylvania Press, 1979), which presents a more balanced contextual view—"neither worshipful nor condemnatory"—of American medicine. Edmund D. Pellegrino's "The Sociocultural Impact of Twentieth-Century Therapeutics" (Vogel and Rosenberg, pp. 245–66) demonstrates persuasively how "the effectiveness of modern treatment raises public expectations" (p. 261) and in doing so further exacerbates the tensions and conflicts inherent in the doctor-patient relationship. Charles E. Rosenberg's *The Care of Strangers: The Rise of America's Hospital System* (New York: Basic Books, Inc., 1987) views the problem of expectations and their effect within the context of the hospital, which Rosenberg sees as a microcosm of American society.

CHAPTER 4

1. Peter L. Berger and Thomas Luckmann, *The Social Construction of Reality: A Treatise in the Sociology of Knowledge* (New York: Doubleday, 1966; Anchor Books edition, 1967), p. 132.

2. Berger and Luckmann, p. 132.

3. Berger and Luckmann, p. 132–33.

4. Berger and Luckmann, p. 137.

5. Berger and Luckmann, p. 138.

6. Berger and Luckmann, p. 141.

7. Berger and Luckmann, p. 147.

8. Clyde Kluckhohn, *Mirror for Man* (New York: McGraw-Hill, 1949), p. 17.

9. Kluckhohn, p. 24.

10. A. L. Kroeber and Clyde Kluckhohn, *Culture: A Critical Review of Concepts and Definitions, Papers of the Peabody Museum of American Archeology and Ethnology*, XLVII, No. 1 (Cambridge, Mass.: Harvard Univ. Press, 1952), 181.

11. Berger and Luckmann, p. 153.

12. Berger and Luckmann, p. 152.

13. Berger and Luckmann, pp. 152–53.

14. Berger and Luckmann, p. 37.

15. Kluckhohn, p. 203.

16. Richard E. Sykes, "American Studies and the Concept of Culture: A Theory and Method," in Robert Meredith, ed., *American Studies: Essays on Theory and Method* (Columbus: Charles E. Merrill, 1968), p. 89.

17. H. D. Laswell, "The Structure and Function of Communication in Society," in Lyman Bryson, ed., *The Communication of Ideas* (New York: Harper, 1948), pp. 37–51.

18. Bernard Berelson, "Communication and Public Opinion," in Wilbur Schramm, ed., *Mass Communications* (Urbana: Univ. of Illinois Press), p. 500. Quoted in Melvin L. DeFleur, *Theories of Mass Communications* (New York: D. McKay, 1966), p. 126.

19. For a useful overview of the state of communications research, see David Manning White, "Mass Communications Research: A View in Perspective," in Lewis Anthony Dexter and David Manning White, eds., *People, Society and Mass Communication* (New York: Free Press of Glencoe, 1964), pp. 521–46. Also of value are Dennis McQuail, *Toward a Sociology of Mass Communication* (London: Collier-Macmillan Publ., 1969) and Walter Weiss, "Effects of the Mass Media of Communication," in Gardner Lindzey and Elliot Aronson, eds., *The Handbook of Social Psychology*, Vol. 5, 2nd. ed. (Reading, Mass.: Addison-Wesley Publ. Co., 1969), pp. 77–195.

20. Wilbur Schramm, "The Effects of Mass Communications: A Review," *Journalism Quarterly*, XXVI, No. 4 (Dec. 1949), 397.

21. Joseph T. Klapper, *The Effects of Mass Communications* (Glencoe, Ill: The Free Press, 1960), p. 3.

22. For a useful sampling of more recent work generated by the continuing concern with and study of media artifacts and their effects, see Ben Bagdikian, *The Media Monopoly* (Boston: Beacon Press, 1983); Daniel J. Czitrom, *Media and the American Mind: From Morse to McLuhan* (Chapel Hill: Univ. of North Carolina Press, 1982); W. Phillips Davison et al., *Mass Media: Systems and Effects* (New York: Praeger, 1976); and Dennis McQuail, *Mass Communications Theory: An Introduction* (London: Sage, 1983).

23. See Klapper, pp. 50–52.

24. Weiss, pp. 115–16. Elaborating on Weiss is another view of media effects, one that asks not what media do to people but rather what people do with the media: see Karl E. Rosengren et al., eds., *Media Gratifications Research: Current Perspectives* (London: Sage, 1985).

25. This is a necessary generalization. Obviously, there have always been groups of people with little or no access to or hope for adequate medical care. Their situation

is all the more difficult, for they, too, are socialized to heightened expectations about doctors even though their own experiences contradict the idealized image.

26. See John C. Burnham, "American Medicine's Golden Age: What Happened to It?" *Science*, 215 (March 19, 1982), 1474–79; Paul Starr, *The Social Transformation of American Medicine* (New York: Basic Books, Inc., 1982); and Morris J. Vogel and Charles E. Rosenberg, eds., *The Therapeutic Revolution: Essays in the Social History of American Medicine* (Philadelphia: Univ. of Pennsylvania Press, 1979).

CHAPTER 5

1. Evelyn Rivers Wilbanks, "The Physician in the American Novel, 1870–1955," *Bulletin of Bibliography*, XXII, vii (Sept.–Dec. 1958), p. 164.

2. Lois Elizabeth DeBakey, "The Physician-scientist as Character in Nineteenth-Century American Literature," diss., Tulane Univ., 1963, p. 1.

3. DeBakey, p. 313.

4. William M. Marchand, "The Changing Role of the Medical Doctor in Selected Plays in American Drama," diss., Univ. of Minnesota, 1966, p. 208.

5. See Evelyn Rivers Wilbanks, "The Doctor as Romantic Hero," and Nancy Y. Hoffman, "The Doctor as Scapegoat: A Study in Ambivalence," *Journal of the American Medical Association*, Vol. 220, No. 1 (April 3, 1972) 54–57 and 58–61. Also see Martha Banta, "Changing Attitudes Toward the Doctor in American Literature," *University of Washington Medicine*, Vol. 7, No. 4 (Winter 1980), 11–18; John A. Cameron, "The Image of the Physician in the American Novel, 1859–1925," Ann Arbor, Mich.: Xerox University Microfilms, 1973; Robert A. Kimbrough, M.D., "Physicians in Current Fiction," *American Journal of Obstetrics and Gynecology*, Vol. LXV (March 1953) 472–78; Carolyn B. Norris, "The Image of Physicians in Modern American Literature," Ann Arbor, Mich.: University Microfilms International, 1969; and David Edward Stooke, "The Portrait of the Physician in Selected Prose Fiction of Nineteenth-Century American Authors," Ann Arbor, Mich.: Xerox University Microfilms, 1976.

6. One minor exception is Dr. Stevens, the narrator of Charles Brockden Brown's *Arthur Mervyn* (1799–1800). Brown uses Stevens' benignity and professional stature to lend credence to the tale told by the book's title character. Although set in Philadelphia during the yellow fever epidemic of 1793, the novel uses both the plague and the physician-narrator merely as framing devices.

7. Nathaniel Hawthorne, "Ethan Brand," in *Nathaniel Hawthorne: Selected Tales and Sketches* (New York: Holt, Rinehart and Winston, 1963), p. 305. Subsequent references are indicated parenthetically.

8. Nathaniel Hawthorne, "The Birthmark," in *Selected Tales*, p. 208. Subsequent references are indicated parenthetically.

9. Nathaniel Hawthorne, "Rappaccini's Daughter," in *Selected Tales*, p. 269. Subsequent references are indicated parenthetically.

10. Hawthorne presents this explicit description of the setting most appropriate for a romance-writer to use in "The Custom House" section of *The Scarlet Letter*. The technique and its attendant ambiguities and alternative interpretations are a crucial device in and a hallmark of Hawthorne's fiction.

11. Nathaniel Hawthorne, *The Scarlet Letter*, Larzer Ziff, ed. (New York: Bobbs-Merrill, 1963), pp. 113–14. Subsequent references are indicated parenthetically.

12. Hawthorne continues to explore the relationship between expertise and a person's potential for evil in *Dr. Grimshawe's Secret* and in three other fragments of novels he left unfinished at his death. Never again, though, would he give such an eloquent rendering of the issue as he does in *The Scarlet Letter*.

13. Oliver Wendell Holmes, *Elsie Venner*, Vol. V of *The Works of Oliver Wendell Holmes* (Boston: Houghton, Mifflin Co., 1891), p. vii. Subsequent references are indicated parenthetically.

14. Oliver Wendell Holmes, *The Guardian Angel*, Vol. VI of *The Works of Oliver Wendell Holmes* (Boston: Houghton, Mifflin Co., 1892).

15. Oliver Wendell Holmes, *A Mortal Antipathy*, Vol. VII of *The Works of Oliver Wendell Holmes* (Boston: Houghton, Mifflin Co., 1892).

16. S. Weir Mitchell, *In War Time* (New York: The Century Company, 1903), p. 3. Subsequent references are indicated parenthetically.

17. S. Weir Mitchell, *Characteristics* (New York: The Century Company, 1903), p. 1. Subsequent references are indicated parenthetically.

18. S. Weir Mitchell, *Dr. North and His Friends* (New York: The Century Company, 1903), p. 456. Subsequent references are indicated parenthetically.

19. S. Weir Mitchell, *Circumstance* (New York: The Century Company, 1903), p. 42. Subsequent references are indicated parenthetically.

20. William Dean Howells, *Dr. Breen's Practice* (Boston: Houghton, Mifflin Co., 1881), p. 12. Subsequent references are indicated parenthetically.

21. Sarah Orne Jewett, *A Country Doctor* (Boston: Houghton, Mifflin Co., 1884; republished in 1970 by Literature House/Gregg Press, Upper Saddle River, N.J.), pp. 32–33. Subsequent references are indicated in text.

CHAPTER 6

1. George Washington Cable, *Dr. Sevier* (New York: Scribner's Sons, 1887), p. 6. Subsequent references are indicated parenthetically.

2. Mary E. Wilkins-Freeman, *Doc Gordon* (New York: The Authors and Newspapers Association, 1906), p. 31. Subsequent references are indicated parenthetically.

3. Joseph C. Lincoln, *Dr. Nye of North Ostable* (New York: Appleton and Co., 1923). Subsequent references are indicated parenthetically.

4. George J. Zaffiras, *The Doctor From Iowa* (New York: Beechurst Press, 1949), p. 31. Subsequent references are indicated parenthetically.

5. Robert Herrick, *The Web of Life* (New York: Garrett Press, reprint of the first edition, 1970), p. 9. Subsequent references are indicated parenthetically.

6. Herrick continued to explore the relationship between wealth and altruism, and particularly the tension between genuine healing and financial success in *The Master of the Inn* (1908) and *The Healer* (1911). Despite their popularity—the former went through eighteen printings and the latter formed the basis for a 1935 film—neither book is as well written as *The Web of Life*.

7. John Steinbeck, *In Dubious Battle* (New York: Covici Friede, 1936), p. 143.

8. Carson McCullers, *The Heart Is A Lonely Hunter* (Boston: Houghton, Mifflin Co., 1940).

9. John O'Hara, *A Family Party* (New York: Random House, 1956), p. 3. Subsequent references are indicated parenthetically.

10. Gerald Green, *The Last Angry Man* (New York: Scribner's Sons, 1956), p. 1. Subsequent references are indicated parenthetically.

11. Henry James, *The Wings of the Dove* (New York: The Modern Library, n. d.), p. 95. Subsequent references are indicated parenthetically.

12. In this echo of Melville's "Bartleby, the Scrivener," James may be hinting at the incomprehensible futility (and odd nobility) of Milly Theale's self-destruction. Another possible hint, and one that would be characteristic of James's verbal playfulness, is evident in the very naming of his heroine. Milly Theale is, quite simply, not a dove; rather she is a teal, a short-necked river duck indigenous to Europe and America.

13. Sherwood Anderson, *Winesburg, Ohio* (New York: The Viking Press, 1960), p. [v]. Subsequent references are indicated parenthetically.

14. F. Scott Fitzgerald, *Tender is the Night* (London: The Bodley Head Press, 1964, reprint of the 1934 Scribner's edition), p. 81. Subsequent references are indicated parenthetically.

15. William Faulkner, *The Wild Palms* (New York: Random House, 1939). Subsequent references are indicated parenthetically.

16. Alice Payne Hackett, *Seventy Years of Best Sellers* (New York: R. R. Bowker Co., 1967), p. 2.

17. Hackett herself notes that the term "best-seller" is a comparative one, and she takes care to use it to describe "not necessarily the best books, but the books that people liked best." I have relied on her compilations, based as they are on *Publisher's Weekly's* annual best-seller lists (which took over *The Bookman's* compilations in 1912) because these lists by design do *not* include book club sales or paperback reprint editions. They are intended to show as accurately as possible the reading tastes of bookstore patrons, the supposedly more regular buyers of books. Hackett's first edition (1946) listed only the "overall best-sellers" from 1895–1945. Her two subsequent editions, following the rise of the inexpensive paperback, expanded the scope to include combined sales, hardbound only sales, and paperback only sales (Hackett, p. 4).

18. Frank Luther Mott, in *Golden Multitudes: The Story of Best-Sellers in the United States* (New York: Macmillan, 1947), allows best-seller status to a book achieving a total *all-time* sale equal to 1 percent of the nation's population in the decade in which the book was published. Mott's variable criterion would denote *The Scarlet Letter* as a best-seller while denying the accolade to all but two of the novels (*Magnificent Obsession* and *Not As A Stranger*) on Hackett's list.

19. Mott asserts that "there is no formula which may be depended upon to produce a best-seller" (p. 285), although he is willing to grant that the study of best-sellers "may be rewarding" to writers and publishers, as well as "to sociologists and historians" (p. 291). A more systematic view is advanced by John Harvey in "The Content Characteristics of Best-Selling Novels," *Public Opinion Quarterly*, XVII, i (Spring 1953), 91–114. Harvey points out that "certain content variables do appear to be associated with sales figures" (p. 91). After presenting his generalized list of these content characteristics (sentimentality, sensationalism, a predominance of unhappiness and anger, readability, the portrayal of contemporary events, and so on), Harvey goes on to speak about the complexity of causal factors contributing to the sale of best-sellers. He concludes by negating the possibility of fully describing

those factors while asserting that the correlative factors he has already listed clearly suggest "avenues of approach to the problem" (p. 114).

20. James D. Hart, *The Popular Book* (New York: Oxford Univ. Press, 1950), p. 285.

21. Ralph Connor, *The Doctor* (New York: Fleming H. Revell Co., 1906), p. 40. Subsequent references are indicated parenthetically.

22. Sinclair Lewis, *Main Street* (New York: New American Library, 1962, originally published in 1920), p. 14. Subsequent references are indicated parenthetically.

23. F. B. Young, "The Doctor in Literature," *Essays By Divers Hands* (The Transactions of the Royal Society of Literature of the United Kingdom), New Series, XV (London: Oxford Univ. Press, 1936), p. 33. Also see G. Edmund Gifford, Jr., M.D., "Fildes and 'The Doctor,' " *JAMA*, Vol. 224, n. 1 (April 2, 1973), 61–63.

24. Mark Schorer, "Afterword" to *Arrowsmith* (New York: New American Library, 1961), pp. 431–438.

25. Sinclair Lewis, *Arrowsmith* (New York: New American Library, 1961, originally published in 1925), p. 45. Subsequent references are indicated parenthetically.

26. Hackett, p. 14. Other medical best-sellers that have sold over one million copies in all editions are *Not As A Stranger* (2,667,977), *The Wild Palms* (1,503,600), *The Interns* (1,126,365), and *Spencer Brade, M.D.* (1,017,351).

27. *Book Review Digest* [Books of 1930], Vol. 26 (New York: The H. W. Wilson Co., 1931), p. 291.

28. Lloyd C. Douglas, *Magnificent Obsession* (New York: Pocket Books, 1973 printing), pp. 144—145. Subsequent references are indicated parenthetically.

29. Mary Roberts Rinehart, *My Story: A New Edition and Seventeen New Years* (New York: Rinehart & Co., 1948, original edition published in 1931), p. 89. Subsequent references are indicated parenthetically.

30. Mary Roberts Rinehart, *The Doctor* (New York: Farrar and Rinehart, 1935), p. 4. Subsequent references are indicated parenthetically.

31. *The Social System* (Glencoe, Ill.: The Free Press, 1951), pp. 458–462. Also see George Montiero, "The Limits of Professionalism: A Sociological Approach to Faulkner, Fitzgerald and Hemingway," *Criticism*, XV, 2 (Spring 1973), 145–155 for a discussion of how the failure to maintain the needed detachment that affective neutrality makes possible leads to the destruction of both Dick Diver and Harry Wilbourne.

32. Morton Thompson, *Not As A Stranger* (New York: Scribner's Sons, 1954), p. 1. Subsequent references are indicated parenthetically.

33. Howard S. Becker et al., *Boys in White: Student Culture in Medical School* (Chicago: Univ. of Chicago Press, 1961), pp. 107ff.

34. Taylor Caldwell, *Testimony of Two Men* (Greenwich, Conn.: Fawcett Crest, 1969), pp. 660–667. Subsequent references are indicated parenthetically.

CHAPTER 7

1. Raymond Stedman, quoted in Robert Campbell, *The Golden Years of Broadcasting: A Celebration of the First Fifty Years of Radio and TV on NBC* (New York: Scribner's Sons, 1976), p. 153.

2. See Herbert J. Gans, *Popular Culture and High Culture* (New York: Basic Books, Inc., 1974) for a different view of the effect of vicarious experience shared via the media. Gans is skeptical about the effect of "individual" portrayals in any medium and feels that they are "ephemeral for most people." Although likely true that any single product of popular culture would have little long-range effect, the significance of myriad portrayals presented in a continuous stream is likely to be far different, more pervasive, potentially more persuasive.

3. John Tebbel, *The Media in America* (New York: Thomas Y. Crowell, 1974), pp. 248–251. Also see Tebbel's *A History of Book Publishing in the United States, Vol. II: The Expansion of an Industry* (New York: R. R. Bowker Co., 1975), pp. 481ff.

4. Charles A. Madison, "Current Trends in American Publishing," in Kathryn Luther Henderson, ed., *Trends in American Publishing* (Champaign: Univ. of Illinois Graduate School of Library Science, 1968), p. 18.

5. Charles A. Madison, *Book Publishing in America* (New York: McGraw-Hill, 1966), p. 548. Also see Roland Marchand, *Advertising The American Dream: Making Way for Modernity, 1920–1940* (Berkeley: Univ. of California Press, 1985).

6. Frank Gruber, *The Pulp Jungle* (Los Angeles: Sherbourne Press, 1967), p. 114.

7. Max Brand, *The Secret of Dr. Kildare* (New York: Beagle Books, 1972, copyright 1931), p. 1.

8. "Talk With the Author," *Newsweek*, 57, n. 3 (Jan. 16, 1961), 82.

9. Frank G. Slaughter, "Elements of Successful Novel Writing," *The Writer*, 85, n. 4 (Apr. 1972), 18–19.

10. Frank G. Slaughter, "When Scalpel Sharpens Pen," *The Writer*, 81, n. 7 (July 1968), 17.

11. Frank G. Slaughter, *That None Should Die* (New York: Pocket Books, 1972, copyright 1941), p. 387.

12. Frank G. Slaughter, *Spencer Brade, M.D.* (New York: Pocket Books, 1973, copyright 1942), p. 80.

13. Benjamin Siegel, *Doctors and Wives* (New York: Dell Publ. Co., 1970); Dorothy Dawes, *Resort M.D.* (New York: Ace Books, 1975); Suzanne Jaffe, *Cruise Ship M.D.* (New York: Ace Books, 1975); and Milton R. Bass, *The Doctor Who Made House Calls* (New York: Dell Publ. Co., 1973).

14. James Kerr, *The Clinic* (Greenwich, Conn.: Fawcett Publ., 1968); Eleazar Lipsky, *Malpractice* (New York: Warner Books, 1972); Paige Mitchell, *A Wilderness of Monkeys* (New York: Popular Library, 1965); and Noah Gordon, *The Death Committee* (Greenwich, Conn.: Fawcett Publ., 1969).

15. Kate Wilhelm, *The Clewiston Test* (New York: Pocket Books, 1977); Henry Denker, *The Experiment* (New York: Pocket Books, 1977); Michael Crichton, *The Terminal Man* (New York: Bantam Books, 1973); and Ronald J. Glasser, M.D., *Ward 402* (New York: Pocket Books, 1974).

16. Irwin Philip Sobel, *The Hospital Makers* (Greenwich, Conn.: Fawcett Publ., 1974); Benjamin Siegel, *Four Doctors* (New York: Dell Publ. Co., 1976); Richard Frede, *The Interns* (New York: Random House, 1960); and Dr. X, *Intern* (Greenwich, Conn.: Fawcett Publ., 1965).

17. Robin Cook, *Coma* (New York: New American Library, 1977); *Brain* (New York: New American Library, 1981); *Fever* (New York: New American Library, 1982); *Godplayer* (New York: New American Library, 1983); *Mindbend* (New

York: New American Library, 1985). Also see Michael Palmer, *Side Effects* (New York: Bantam Books, 1985); Leslie Ann Horvitz and H. Harris Gerhard, M.D., *The Donors* (New York: New American Library, 1982); David Osborn, *Heads* (New York: Bantam Books, 1985); and Mary Higgins Clark, *The Cradle Will Fall* (New York: Dell Publ. Co., 1980).

CHAPTER 8

1. Giraud Chester et al., *Television and Radio* (New York: Appleton-Century Crofts, 1973), p. v. See also Mark S. Hoffman, ed., *The World Almanac and Book of Facts 1987* (New York: Pharos Books, 1987), p. 373, and Otto Johnson, ed., *Information Please Almanac, Atlas and Yearbook 1987* (Boston: Houghton, Mifflin Co., 1987), pp. 726–728.

2. George Gerbner and Larry Gross, "The Scary World of TV's Heavy Viewer," *Psychology Today*, IX (April 1976), 42.

3. Harry M. Brown, "TV and the American Way of Life," in James C. Austin, ed. *Popular Literature in America* (Bowling Green, Ohio: Bowling Green Univ. Press, 1972), pp. 200–201.

4. Melvin L. DeFleur, "Occupational Roles as Portrayed on Television," *Public Opinion Quarterly*, XXVIII, 1 (Spring 1964), 74.

5. Rose K. Goldsen, *The Show and Tell Machine* (New York: The Dial Press, 1977), p. 14. See the appendix to Chapter 1 for readings on the effects of "controlling visual materials and discourse in the social environment" (p. 292).

6. "Medical Center" (CBS-TV), March 18, 1970; "Medical Center" (CBS-TV), March 11, 1970; "Medical Center" (CBS-TV), Feb. 4, 1970; "St. Elsewhere" (NBC-TV), Jan. 18, 1983.

7. Gerbner and Gross, p. 44. Also see Michael Real's discussion of Welby in *Mass-Mediated Culture* (Englewood Cliffs, N.J.: Prentice-Hall, Inc., 1977).

8. Walter Weiss, "Effects of the Mass Media of Communication," in Gardner Lindzey and Elliot Aronson, eds., *The Handbook of Social Psychology*, Vol. 5, 2nd ed. (Reading, Mass.: Addison-Wesley Publ. Co., 1969), p. 112. Also see Robert S. Alley, "Medical Melodrama," in Brian G. Rose, ed., *TV Genres: A Handbook and Reference Guide* (Westport, Conn.: Greenwood Press, 1985), pp. 73–89.

9. A newer incarnation of television's medical idealization is *"Buck James"* whose title character is portrayed by Dennis Weaver, who had played the deputy Chester on the long-running *"Gunsmoke"* (1955–64) and who took the title role of *"McCloud"* (1970–77), a modernized deputy marshall transplanted to New York City. As the surgeon Buck James, Weaver mixes his western background with familiar medical melodrama in altogether predictable ways.

Bibliography

This bibliography is more comprehensive than are the textual notes. As is often the case, many useful materials provided background and context for this study without finding their way, explicitly, into the notes.

PRIMARY SOURCES

Anderson, Sherwood. *Winesburg, Ohio*. New York: The Viking Press, 1960.
Bass, Milton. *The Doctor Who Made House Calls*. New York: Dell Publ. Co., 1973.
Brand, Max. *Calling Dr. Kildare*. 1942; rpt. New York: Beagle Books, 1972.
———. *Dr. Kildare Takes Charge*. 1941; rpt. New York: Beagle Books, 1972.
———. *Dr. Kildare's Crisis*. 1942; rpt. New York: Beagle Books, 1972.
———. *Dr. Kildare's Search* and *Dr. Kildare's Hardest Case*. 1943; rpt. New York: Beagle Books, 1971.
———. *Dr. Kildare's Trial*. 1942; rpt. New York: Beagle Books, 1972.
———. *The Secret of Dr. Kildare*. 1936; rpt. New York: Beagle Books, 1972.
———. *Young Dr. Kildare*. 1941; rpt. New York: Beagle Books, 1971.
Broughton, Rhoda. *Dr. Cupid*. Philadelphia: 1886.
Brown, Charles Brockden. *Arthur Mervyn; or Memoirs of the Year 1793*. Philadelphia: McKay, 1889.
Burnham, Clara Louise. *Dr. Latimer*. New York: 1893.
Cable, George Washington. *Dr. Sevier*. New York: Scribner's Sons, 1910.
Caldwell, Taylor. *Testimony of Two Men*. Greenwich, Conn. Fawcett Crest, 1969.
Clark, Eleanor. *Dr. Heart: A Novella and Other Stories*. New York: Pantheon Books, 1974.
Clark, Mary Higgins. *The Cradle Will Fall*. New York: Dell Publ. Co., 1980.
Connor, Ralph. *The Doctor*. New York: Fleming H. Revell Co., 1906.
Cook, Robin. *Brain*. New York: New American Library, 1981.
———. *Coma*. New York: New American Library, 1977.
———. *Fever*. New York: New American Library, 1982.

——. *Godplayer*. New York: New American Library, 1983.

——. *Mindbend*. New York: New American Library, 1985.

Cooper, Irving S., M.D. *The Victim is Always the Same*. New York: Harper & Row, 1970.

Crichton, Michael. *Five Patients*. New York: Bantam Books, 1971.

——. *The Terminal Man*. New York: Bantam Books, 1973.

Dawes, Dorothy. *Resort M.D.* New York: Ace Books, 1975.

Denker, Henry. *The Experiment*. New York: Pocket Books, 1977.

Douglas, Diana. *Doctor in Shadow*. New York: New American Library, 1967.

Douglas, Lloyd C. *Doctor Hudson's Secret Journal*. New York: Grosset & Dunlap, 1939.

——. *Magnificent Obsession*. New York: Grosset & Dunlap, 1929.

Fabricant, Noah D. and Heinz Werner, eds. *A Treasury of Doctor Stories By the World's Great Authors*. New York: Frederick Fell, 1946.

Faulkner, William. *The Wild Palms*. New York: Random House, 1939.

Fitzgerald, F. Scott. *Tender Is The Night*. London: The Bodley Head Edition, 1964.

Frede, Richard. *The Interns*. New York: Random House, 1960.

Glasser, Ronald J., M.D. *Ward 402*. New York: Pocket Books, 1974.

Goldberg, Marshall, M.D. *A Deadly Operation*. New York: Pinnacle Books, 1972.

Gordon, Noah. *The Death Committee*. Greenwich, Conn. Fawcett Publ., 1969.

Green, Gerald. *The Hostage Heart*. New York: Playboy Press, 1976.

——. *The Last Angry Man*. New York: Scribner's Sons, 1956.

Hall, James N. *Doctor Dogbody's Leg*. Boston: Little, Brown and Co., 1940.

Hawthorne, Nathaniel. "Dr. Heidegger's Experiment," in *The Complete Novels and Selected Tales of Nathaniel Hawthorne*. New York: The Modern Library, 1956, pp. 945–952.

——. *Dr. Grimshawe's Secret*. Boston: James R. Osgood & Co., 1883.

——. *The Scarlet Letter*. New York: Bobbs-Merrill, 1963.

——. *Selected Tales and Sketches*. New York: Holt, Rinehart, and Winston, 1963.

Henry, Caleb Sprague. *Doctor Oldham*. New York: Appleton & Co., 1860.

Herrick, Robert. *The End of Desire*. New York: Macmillan, 1932.

——. *The Healer*. New York: Macmillan, 1911.

——. *The Master of the Inn*. New York: Scribners Sons, 1908.

——. *The Web of Life*. New York: Macmillan, 1900.

Higgins, Margaret. *A Doctor for the Dead*. New York: Ace Books, 1976.

Holmes, Oliver Wendell. *Elsie Venner*. Boston: Houghton, Mifflin Co., 1892.

——. *The Guardian Angel*. Boston: Houghton, Mifflin Co., 1892.

——. *Medical Essays: 1842–1882*. Boston: Houghton, Mifflin Co., 1892.

——. *A Mortal Antipathy*. Boston: Houghton, Mifflin Co., 1892.

Hooker, Richard. *M*A*S*H*. New York: Pocket Books, 1972.

—— and William E. Butterworth. *M*A*S*H Goes to Hollywood*. New York: Pocket Books, 1976.

——. *M*A*S*H Goes to London*. New York: Pocket Books, 1976.

——. *M*A*S*H Goes to Montreal*. New York: Pocket Books, 1977.

Horvitz, Leslie Alan and H. Harris Gerhard, M.D. *The Donors*. New York: New American Library, 1982.

Howells, William Dean. *Dr. Breen's Practice*. Boston: Houghton, Mifflin Co., 1881.

Jaffee, Suzanne. *Cruise Ship M.D.* New York: Ace Books, 1975.

James, Henry. *Wings of the Dove*. 1902; rpt. New York: The Modern Library, n.d.

Jewett, Sarah Orne. *A Country Doctor*. Boston: Houghton, Mifflin Co., 1884.

Johnston, William. *Medical Story #2: Kill Me Please*... New York: New American Library, 1976.

Kappelman, Murray, M.D. *The Child Healers*. New York: Dell Publ. Co., 1971.

Kerr, James. *The Clinic*. Greenwich, Conn.: Fawcett Publ., 1968.

Lewis, Sinclair. *Arrowsmith*. New York: New American Library, 1953.

———. *Main Street*. New York: New American Library, 1962.

Lincoln, Joseph C. *Doctor Nye of North Ostable*. New York: Appleton & Co., 1923.

Lipsky, Eleazar. *Malpractice*. New York: Warner Books, 1977.

McCullers, Carson. *The Heart Is A Lonely Hunter*. Boston: Houghton, Mifflin Co., 1940.

MacKenzie, Rachael. *RISK*. New York: The Viking Press, 1970.

Mitchell, Paige. *A Wilderness of Monkeys*. New York: Popular Library, 1965.

Mitchell, S. Weir. *"The Autobiography of a Quack" and Other Stories*. New York: The Century Co., 1901.

———. *Characteristics*. New York: The Century Co., 1915.

———. *Circumstance*. New York: The Century Co., 1903.

———. *Dr. North and His Friends*. New York: The Century Co., 1915.

———. *In War Time*. New York: The Century Co., 1910.

Nolen, William A., M.D. *The Making of a Surgeon*. New York: Pocket Books, 1970.

———. *A Surgeon's World*. Greenwich, Conn.: Fawcett Publ., 1974.

O'Hara, John. *A Family Party*. New York: Random House, 1956.

Osborn, David. *Heads*. New York: Bantam Books, 1985.

Palmer, Michael. *Side Effects*. New York: Bantam Books, 1985.

Peters, L. T. *The 11th Plague*. New York: Pinnacle Books, 1973.

Richards, Monty. *Surgeon At Sea*. New York: Belmont Books, 1967.

Rinehart, Mary Roberts. *Breaking Point*. New York: Farrar and Rinehart, 1922.

———. *The Doctor*. New York: Farrar and Rinehart, 1935.

———. *My Story: A New Edition and Seventeen New Years*. New York: Rinehart & Co., 1948.

Rosten, Leo. *Captain Newman, M.D.* London: Victor Gollancz Ltd., 1961.

Rubin, Theodore Isaac, M.D., *Emergency Room Diary*. New York: Bantam Books, 1975.

———. *Shrink!* New York: Popular Library, 1974.

Seifert, Elizabeth. *Army Doctor*. New York: Dodd, Mead, 1942.

———. *Bachelor Doctor*. New York: Dodd, Mead, 1969.

———. *Doctor at the Crossroads*. New York: Dodd, Mead, 1957.

———. *The Doctor Disagrees*. New York: Dodd, Mead, 1953.

———. *Doctor in Love*. New York: Dodd, Mead, 1974.

———. *Doctor in the Family*. New York: Dodd, Mead, 1955.

———. *Dr. Jeremy's Wife*. New York: Dodd, Mead, 1961.

———. *The Doctor Makes A Choice*. New York: Dodd, Mead, 1961.

———. *Doctor Mollie*. New York: Dodd, Mead, 1951; published as *Miss Doctor* in 1952.

———. *Doctor Samaritan*. New York: Dodd, Mead, 1965.

———. *The Doctor's Affair*. New York: Dodd, Mead, 1975.

——. *The Doctor's Bride*. New York: Dodd, Mead, 1960.

——. *The Doctor's Confession*. New York: Dodd, Mead, 1968.

——. *The Doctor's Daughter*. New York: Signet, 1975.

——. *The Doctor's Desperate Hour*. Boston: Hall, 1976.

——. *The Doctor's Kingdom*. New York: Signet, 1974.

——. *The Doctor's Private Life*. Boston: Hall, 1974.

——. *The Doctor's Reputation*. South Yarmouth, Mass.: Curley, 1976.

——. *The Doctor's Strange Secret*. New York: Dodd, Mead, 1962.

——. *The Doctor's Two Lives*. South Yarmouth, Mass.: Curley, 1976.

——. *The Doctor's Two Loves*. New York: Dodd, Mead, 1982.

——. *For Love of a Doctor*. South Yarmouth, Mass.: Curley, 1976.

——. *Four Doctors, Four Wives*. New York: Dodd, Mead, 1975.

——. *Girl Intern*. New York: Dodd, Mead, 1944.

——. *Hegerty, M.D.* New York: Dodd, Mead, 1966.

——. *Hillbilly Doctor*. New York: Dodd, Mead, 1940.

——. *The Honor of Doctor Shelton*. New York: Dodd, Mead, 1962.

——. *The Rival Doctors*. New York: Dodd, Mead, 1967.

——. *Two Doctors and a Girl*. New York: Dodd, Mead, 1976.

——. *The Two Faces of Dr. Collier*. New York: Signet, 1974.

——. *Young Doctor Galahad*. New York: Dodd, Mead, 1938.

Siegel, Benjamin. *Doctors and Wives*. New York: Dell, 1977.

——. *Four Doctors*. New York: Dell, 1975.

Slaughter, Frank G. *Air Surgeon*. New York: Doubleday, 1943.

——. *Battle Surgeon*. New York: Pocket Books, 1976.

——. *Code Five*. New York: Pocket Books, 1972.

——. *Convention M.D.* New York: Pocket Books, 1973.

——. *Countdown*. New York: Doubleday, 1970.

——. *Daybreak*. New York: Doubleday, 1958.

——. *Divine Mistress*. New York: Pocket Books, 1975.

——. *East Side General*. New York: Doubleday, 1952.

——. *Epidemic*. New York: Doubleday, 1961.

——. *The Healer*. New York: Pocket Books, 1974.

——. *In a Dark Garden*. New York: Pocket Books, 1976.

——. *Plaque Ship*. New York: Pocket Books, 1977.

——. *A Savage Place*. New York: Pocket Books, 1972.

——. *Spencer Brade, M.D.* New York: Pocket Books, 1973.

——. *Surgeon, U. S. A.* New York: Pocket Books, 1973.

——. *Surgeon's Choice*. New York: Doubleday, 1969.

——. *Sword and Scalpel*. New York: Pocket Books, 1976.

——. *That None Should Die*. New York: Pocket Books, 1972.

——. *Tomorrow's Miracle*. New York: Doubleday, 1962.

——. *Women in White*. New York: Pocket Books, 1975.

Sobel, Irwin Philip, M.D. *The Hospital Makers*. Greenwich, Conn.: Fawcett Publ., 1973.

Steinbeck, John. *In Dubious Battle*. New York: Covici Friede, 1936.

Thompson, Morton. *Not As A Stranger*. New York: Scribner's Sons, 1955.

Ward, Elizabeth Stuart Phelps. *Dr. Zay*. Boston: 1882.

——. *Though Life Us Do Part*. Boston: 1908.

Ward, Mary Jane. *The Snake Pit*. New York: Random House, 1946.

Wilhelm, Kate. *The Clewiston Test*. New York: Pocket Books, 1977.

Wilkins-Freeman, Mary E. *Doc Gordon*. New York: Authors and Newspapers Association, 1906.

Woolfolk, William. *the president's doctor*[sic]. New York: Playboy Press, 1975.

X, Dr. *Intern*. Greenwich, Conn.: Fawcett Crest, 1965.

Zaffiras, George J. *The Doctor From Iowa*. New York: Beechhurst Press, 1949.

SECONDARY SOURCES

Ackerknecht, Erwin H., M.D. "On the Teaching of Medical History," in Iago Galdston, M.D., ed. *On the Utility of Medical History*. New York: International Universities Press, Inc., 1957.

————. *A Short History of Medicine*. New York: The Ronald Press, 1968.

Alley, Robert. S. "Medical Melodrama," in Brian G. Rose, ed., *TV Genres: A Handbook and Reference Guide*. Westport, Conn.: Greenwood Press, 1985, pp. 73–89.

American Medical Association. *Horizons Unlimited*. Chicago: American Medical Association, 1966.

Anderson, Fred. "The Growing Pains of Medical Care," *The New Republic*. Jan. 17, 24 and Feb. 7, 1970.

Andrews, William, F. R. H. S., ed. *The Doctor in History, Literature, Folk-lore, etc.* London: Simpkin, Marshall, Hamilton, Kent & Co., 1896.

Arlen, Michael. *The View From Highway 1*. New York: Ballantine Books, 1977.

Arnheim, R. "The World of the Daytime Serial," in P. F. Lazarsfeld and F. N. Stanton, eds. *Radio Research 1942–1943*. New York: Duell, Sloan, and Pearce, 1944.

Austin, James C., ed. *Popular Literature in America*. Bowling Green, Ohio: Bowling Green Univ. Popular Press, 1972.

Bagdikian, Ben. *The Media Monopoly*. Boston: Beacon Press, 1983.

Bailis, Stanley. "The Social Sciences in American Studies: An Integrative Conception." *AQ*, XXVI, 3 (Aug. 1974), 202–224.

Barber, Bernard. "Some Problems in the Sociology of the Professions." *Daedalus*. 92, 4 (Fall 1963), 669–688.

Basalla, George. "Pop Science: The Depiction of Science in Popular Culture," in G. Holton and W. A. Blanpied, eds., *Science and Its Public*. Dodrecht, Holland: D. Reidel Publ. Co., 1976, pp. 261–278.

Becker, Howard S., Blanche Geer, Everett C. Hughes, and Anselm Strauss. *Boys in White: Student Culture in Medical School*. Chicago: Univ. of Chicago Press, 1961.

Bell, Daniel, ed. *Toward the Year 2000: Work in Progress*. Boston: Houghton, Mifflin Co., 1968.

Berelson, Bernard. *Content Analysis in Communication Research*. Glencoe, Ill.: The Free Press, 1952.

Berger, Peter L. and Thomas Luckmann. *The Social Construction of Reality*. New York: Doubleday, 1966; Anchor Books Edition, 1967.

Bledstein, Burton J. *The Culture of Professionalism: The Middle Class and the Development of Higher Education in America*. New York: W. W. Norton, 1976.

Bloom, Samuel W. *The Doctor and His Patient*. New York: The Free Press, 1965.

Blumer, Herbert. *Movies and Conduct*. New York: Macmillan, 1933.

Blumhagen, Dan W. "The Doctors' White Coat: The Image of the Physician in Modern America," *Annals of Internal Medicine*, 91, 1 (July 1979), 111–116.

Bowron, Bernard, Leo Marx, and Arnold Rose. "Literature and Covert Culture," in Joseph K. Kwiat and Mary C. Turpie, eds., *Studies in American Culture*. Minneapolis: Univ. of Minnesota Press, 1960, pp. 84–95.

Brooks, Tim and Earle Marsh. *The Complete Directory to Prime Time Network TV Shows 1946-Present*, rev. ed. New York: Ballantine Books, 1981.

Bullough, Vern L. *The Development of Medicine as a Profession*. New York: Hofner Publ. Co., 1966.

Burnham, John. C. "American Medicine's Golden Age: What Happened to It?" *Science*, 215 (March 19, 1982), 1474–79.

Cahal, Mac F. "The Image." *JAMA*, 185, 3 (July 20, 1963), 183–187.

Califano, Joseph A., Jr. *America's Health Care Revolution: Who Lives? Who Dies? Who Pays?* New York: Random House, 1987.

Campbell, Robert. *The Golden Years of Broadcasting: A Celebration of the First Fifty Years of Radio and TV on NBC*. New York: Scribner's Sons, 1976.

Carr-Saunders, A. M. and P. A. Wilson. *The Professions*. Oxford: The Clarendon Press, 1933.

Carter, Richard. *The Doctor Business*. New York: Doubleday, 1958.

Cirino, Robert. *Don't Blame the People*. New York: Random House, 1971.

Coan, Otis W. *America in Fiction: An Annotated List of Novels That Interpret Aspects of Life in the United States, Canada, and Mexico*, 5th ed. Palo Alto, Calif.: Pacific Books, 1967.

Coffin, T. "Television's Impact on Society." *American Psychologist*, 10 (1955), 630–41.

Cogan, Morris L. "Toward A Definition of Profession." *Harvard Educational Review*, 23, 1 (Winter 1953), 33–50.

Cook, Fred J. *The Plot Against the Patient*. Englewood Cliffs, N.J.: Prentice-Hall, Inc., 1967.

Cordtz, Dan. "Change Begins in the Doctor's Office." *Fortune*, 81 (Jan. 1970), 84ff.

Crichton, Michael. "The High Cost of Cure." *The Atlantic*, 225 (March 1970), 49–57.

"The Crisis in Health Care." *Time*, 95 (March 30, 1976), 54.

Cyclops. "Dr. Welby's Tonic Won't Harm You." *Life*, 10 (May 14, 1971), 18.

Czitrom, Daniel J. *Media and the American Mind: From Morse to McLuhan*. Chapel Hill: Univ. of North Carolina Press, 1982.

Dale, E. *The Content of Motion Pictures*. New York: Macmillan, 1933.

Davidson, Bill. "Another Illness, Another Show." *TV Guide*, 19 (April 24, 1971), 25–28.

———. "Next Week: Periarteritis Nodosa." *TV Guide*, 19 (July 1, 1971), 12–16.

Davidson, Muriel. "Viewer Heal Thyself." *TV Guide*, 21 (July 21, 1973), 21–24.

Davison, W. Phillips, James Boylan and Frederick T. C. Yu. *Mass Media: Systems and Effects*. New York: Praeger Publ., 1976.

DeBakey, Lois Elizabeth. "The Fictional Physician of Nineteenth Century America: Scientific Milieu." *Southern Medical Journal* (Dec. 1966), 1455–63.

————. "The Physician-scientist as Character in Nineteenth Century American Literature." diss., Tulane Univ., 1963.

DeFleur, Melvin L. "Occupational Roles as Portrayed on Television." *Public Opinion Quarterly*, XXVIII, i (Spring 1964), 57–74.

————. *Theories of Mass Communications*. New York: D. McKay, 1966.

Denby, David. "Movies: Documenting America." *The Atlantic*, 225 (March 1970), 139–142.

Dickson, A. T., Jr. *American Historical Fiction*, 3rd. ed. Metuchen, N.J.: The Scarecrow Press, 1971.

Diehl, Digby. "Grandfather Knows Best." *TV Guide*, 18 (June 6, 1970), 24–28.

Duffy, John. *The Healers: The Rise of the Medical Establishment*. New York: McGraw-Hill, 1976.

The Editors of the Yale Law Journal. "The American Medical Association: Power, Purpose, and Politics in Organized Medicine." *The Yale Law Journal*, 63 (May 1954), 938–47.

Edmondson, Madeline and David Rounds. *The Soaps: Daytime Serials of Radio and TV*. New York: Stein and Day, 1973.

Ehrenreich, Barbara and John Ehrenreich. *The American Health Empire: Power, Profits, and Politics*. New York: Random House, 1970.

————and Deirdre English. *Complaints and Disorders: The Sexual Politics of Sickness*. Old Westbury, N.Y.: The Feminist Press (Glass Mountain Pamphlet No. 2), 1973.

————. *Witches, Midwives and Nurses*. Oyster Bay, N.Y.: Glass Mountain Pamphlets, n. d.

Eichelberger, Clayton L. *A Guide to Critical Reviews of United States Fiction, 1870–1910*. Metuchen, N.J.: The Scarecrow Press, 1971.

Emery, P. E. "Psychological Effects of the Western Film: A Study in Television Viewing." *Human Relations*, 12 (1959), 195–231.

Fein, Rashi. *The Doctor Shortage: An Economic Diagnosis*. Washington, D.C.: The Brookings Institute, 1967.

Fishbein, Morris. *A History of the American Medical Association 1847–1947*. Philadelphia: W. B. Saunders Co., 1947.

Freeman, Howard E., Sol Levine, and Leo G. Reeder, eds. *Handbook of Medical Sociology*. Englewood Cliffs, N.J.: Prentice-Hall, Inc., 1963.

Freidson, Eliot. *Patients' Views of Medical Practice*. Chicago: Univ. of Chicago Press, 1980.

————. *Profession of Medicine: A Study of the Sociology of Applied Knowledge*. New York: Harper & Row, 1970.

————. *Professional Dominance: The Social Structure of Medical Care*. New York: Aldine Publ. Co., 1970.

Friedman, Norman. "Studying Film Impact On American Conduct and Culture." *Journal of Popular Film*, III, 2 (Spring 1974), 173–81.

Galdston, Iago, M.D. *The Meaning of Social Medicine*. Cambridge, Mass.: Harvard Univ. Press, 1954.

————, ed. *On the Utility of Medical History*. New York: International Universities Press, Inc., 1957.

Gans, Herbert J. *Popular Culture and High Culture*. New York: Basic Books, Inc., 1974.

Garceau, Oliver. *The Political Life of the American Medical Association*. Hamden, Conn.: Archon Books, 1961.

Geison, Gerald L., ed. *Professions and Professional Ideologies in America*. Chapel Hill: Univ. of North Carolina Press, 1983.

Gerbner, George and Larry Gross. "The Scary World of TV's Heavy Viewer." *Psychology Today*, 9 (April 1976), 41–45.

Gerbner, George, Larry Gross, Michael Morgan, and Nancy Signorielli. "Special Report: Health and Medicine on Television." *The New England Journal of Medicine*, 305, 15 (Oct. 8, 1981), 901–4.

Gifford, Jr., M.D. and G. Edmund. "Fildes and 'The Doctor.' " *JAMA*, 224, 1 (April 2, 1973), 61–63.

Gillman, Neil. Letter to William Safire, quoted in William Safire, "Love That Dare." *New York Times Magazine* (May 17, 1987), p. 12.

Ginzberg, Eli with Miriam Ostow. *Men, Money and Medicine*. New York: Columbia Univ. Press, 1969.

Goldsen, Rose K. *The Show and Tell Machine*. New York: The Dial Press, 1977.

Goode, W. J. "Community Within a Community: The Professions." *American Sociological Review*, 22 (1957), 194–200.

Gross, Martin. *The Doctors*. New York: Random House, 1966.

Gruber, Frank. *The Pulp Jungle*. Los Angeles: Sherbourne Press, 1967.

Hackett, Alice Payne. *70 Years of Best Sellers: 1895–1965*. New York: R. R. Bowker Co., 1967.

Haggard, Howard W. *The Doctor in History*. Freeport, N.Y.: Books for Libraries Press, 1970.

Handel, L. A. *Hollywood Looks At Its Audience*. Urbana: Univ. of Illinois Press, 1950.

Hanley, F. W. and F. Greenburg. "Reflections on the Doctor-Patient Relationship." *Canadian Medical Association Journal*, 86 (June 2, 1962), 1022–24.

Harris, Richard. *A Sacred Trust*. New York: New American Library, 1966.

Hart, James D. *The Popular Book*. New York: Oxford Univ. Press, 1950.

Haskell, Thomas L., ed. *The Authority of Experts: Studies in History and Theory*. Bloomington: Indiana Univ. Press, 1984.

Henderson, Kathryn Luther, ed. *Trends in American Publishing*. Champaign: Univ. of Illinois Graduate School of Library Science, 1968.

Henderson, L. J. "Physician and Patient as a Social System." *The New England Journal of Medicine*, 212, 18 (1935), 821–23.

Hilfiker, David. *Healing the Wounds: A Physician Looks at His Work*. New York: Pantheon Books, 1985.

Hodgson, Godfrey. "The Politics of American Health Care." *The Atlantic*, 232, 4 (Oct. 1973), 45ff.

Hoffman, Mark, ed. *The World Almanac and Book of Facts*. New York: Pharos Books, 1987.

Hoffman, Nancy Y. "The Doctor as Scapegoat: A Study in Ambivalence." *JAMA*, 200, 1 (April 3, 1972), 58–61.

Hovland, C. I. "Effects of the Mass Media of Communication," in G. Lindsey, ed. *Handbook of Social Psychology*. Cambridge, Mass.: Addison-Wesley, 1954, pp. 1062–1103.

"How Good Is Your Doctor?" *Newsweek*, 84 (Dec. 23, 1974), 46–53.

Hudson, Robert P. "Abraham Flexner in Perspective: American Medical Education, 1865–1910," in Judith Walzer Leavitt and Ronald L. Numbers, eds., *Sickness and Health in America*, 2nd ed., rev. Madison: Univ. of Wisconsin Press, 1985, pp. 148–58.

Hughes, Everett C. "Professions." *Daedalus*, 92 (Fall 1963), 655–68.

Illinois University, Davis Lecture Committee. *Essays in the History of Medicine*. Chicago: Univ. of Illinois Press, 1965.

Inter-Professions Conference on Education for Professional Responsibility. *Education for Professional Responsibility*. Pittsburgh: Carnegie Press, 1948.

Jaco, E. Gartly, ed. *Patients, Physicians, and Illness: Sourcebook in Behavioral Science and Medicine*. New York: The Free Press, 1965.

Johnson, Otto, ed. *Information Please Almanac and Yearbook 1987*. Boston: Houghton, Mifflin Co., 1987.

Jones, Anne Hudson. "Medicine and the Physician in Popular Culture," in Inge M. Thomas, ed., *Handbook of American Popular Culture*, Vol. 3. Westport, Conn.: Greenwood Press, 1981.

Jones, Dorothy B. "Quantitative Analysis of Motion Picture Content." *Public Opinion Quarterly*, XIV, 3 (Fall 1950), 554–58.

Josephson, E. M. *Your Life is Their Toy*, 2nd. ed. New York: Chedry Press, 1948.

Kaufman, M. Ralph, M.D. "The Doctor's Image: An Approach to a Study of a Universal Ambivalence." *The Mount Sinai Journal of Medicine*, 43, 1 (Jan.–Feb. 1976), 76–97.

Kaufman, Martin. *American Medical Education: The Formative Years, 1765–1910*. Westport, Conn.: Greenwood Press, 1976.

Katz, Seymour. "Culture and Literature in American Studies." *AQ*, XX, 2, Part 2 (Summer Supplement 1968), 318–29.

Kelly, R. Gordon. "American Children's Literature: An Historiographical Review." *American Literary Realism 1870–1910*, VI (Spring 1973), 89–107.

———. "Literature and the Historian." *AQ*, XXVI, 2 (May 1974), 141–159.

Kennedy, Edward M. *In Critical Condition*. New York: Pocket Books, 1973.

Kett, Joseph F. *The Formation of the American Medical Profession (The Role of Institutions, 1780–1860)*. New Haven: Yale Univ. Press, 1968.

Klapper, Joseph T. *The Effects of Mass Communication*. Glencoe, Ill.: The Free Press, 1960.

Kluckhohn, Clyde. *Mirror for Man*. New York: McGraw-Hill, 1949.

Knowles, John H. "The Balanced Biology of the Teaching Hospital." *The New England Journal of Medicine*, CCLXIX, 8 (Aug. 22, 1963).

———. *Doing Better and Feeling Worse: Health Care in the United States*. New York: W. W. Norton, 1977.

Kolko, Gabriel. *The Triumph of Conservatism*. Chicago: Quadrangle Books, 1967.

Kuklick, Bruce. "Myth and Symbol in American Studies." *AQ*, XVIV, 4 (Oct. 1972), 435–50.

LaGuardia, Robert. *The Wonderful World of TV Soap Operas*. New York: Ballantine Books, 1974.

Lasagna, Louis. *The Doctor's Dilemma*. Freeport, N.Y.: Books for Libraries Press, 1970.

Leavitt, Judith Walzer and Ronald L. Numbers, eds. *Sickness and Health in America*, 2nd ed., rev. Madison: Univ. of Wisconsin Press, 1985.

Lederer, Henry D. "How the Sick View Their World," in E. Gartly Jaco, ed. *Patients, Physicians and Illness: Sourcebook in Behavioral Science and Medicine.* New York: The Free Press, 1965.

Lewis, Roy and Angus Maude. *Professional People.* London: Phoenix House Ltd., 1952.

Lewis, R. W. B. *The American Adam: Innocence, Tragedy and Tradition in the Nineteenth Century.* Chicago: Univ. of Chicago Press (Phoenix Books edition), 1966.

Louis, Sydney and George Agich. "Language and the Physician's Art." *JAMA,* 242, 23 (Dec. 7, 1979), 2580–82.

Lubove, Roy. *The Professional Altruist.* New York: Atheneum, 1969.

Ludmerer, Kenneth M. *Learning to Heal.* New York: Basic Books, Inc., 1985.

McGlothlin, William J. *Patterns of Professional Education.* New York: G. P. Putnam's Sons, 1960.

———. *The Professional Schools.* New York: The Center for Applied Research in Education, 1964.

McQuail, Denis. *Mass Communication Theory: An Introduction.* London: Sage, 1983.

———. *Toward A Sociology of Mass Communication.* London: Collier-McMillan, 1969.

Madison, Charles A. *Book Publishing in America.* New York: McGraw-Hill, 1966.

Marchand, Roland. *Advertising the American Dream: Making Way for Modernity, 1920–1940.* Berkeley: Univ. of California Press, 1985.

Marchand, William M. "The Changing Role of the Medical Doctor in Selected Plays in American Drama." diss., Univ. of Minnesota, 1966.

Marx, Leo. "American Studies—In Defense of an Unscientific Method." *New Literary History,* I, 1 (Oct. 1969), 75–90.

Means, James Howard. "Homo Medicus Americanus." *Daedalus,* 92 (Fall 1963), 701–23.

Mecklin, John M. "Hospitals Need Management Even More Than Money." *Fortune,* 81 (Jan. 1970), 96 ff.

Mendelsohn, Everett, Judith P. Swazey, and Irene Taviss, eds. *Human Aspects of Biomedical Innovation.* Cambridge, Mass.: Harvard Univ. Press, 1971.

Menke, Wayne G. "The Doctor: Change and Conflict in American Medical Practice." diss., Univ. of Minnesota, 1961.

Merton, Robert K., George G. Reader, M.D., and Patricia Kendall, eds. *The Student Physician: Introductory Studies in the Sociology of Medical Education.* Cambridge, Mass.: Harvard Univ. Press, 1957.

Meyers, Harold B. "The Medical-Industrial Complex." *Fortune,* 81 (Jan. 1970), 90ff.

Michelfelder, William. *It's Cheaper To Die.* New York: George Braziller, 1960.

Millerson, Geoffrey. *The Qualifying Associations: A Study in Professionalization.* London: Routledge & Kegan Paul, 1964.

Montiero, George. "The Limits of Professionalism: A Sociological Approach to Faulkner, Fitzgerald, and Hemingway." *Criticism,* XV, 2 (Spring 1973), 145–55.

Morantz-Sanchez, Regina Markell. *Sympathy and Science: Women Physicians in American Medicine.* New York: Oxford Univ. Press, 1987.

Mott, Frank Luther. *Golden Multitudes: The Story of Best Sellers in the United States*. New York: Macmillan, 1947.

Myerhoff, Barbara G. and William R. Larson. "The Doctor as Culture Hero: The Routinization of Charisma." *Human Organization*, 24 (1964), 188–91.

Newcomb, Horace, ed. *Television: The Critical View*. New York: Oxford Univ. Press, 1976.

Norwood, William Frederick. *Medical Education in the United States Before the Civil War*. Philadelphia: Univ. of Pennsylvania Press, 1944.

Parsons, Talcott. *Essays in Sociological Theory*. rev. ed. New York: The Free Press, 1954.

———. *The Social System*. Glencoe, Ill.: The Free Press, 1951.

Podolsky, Edward. "Excerpts from Literature Illustrative of the Popular Distrust of the Medical Profession." *Illinois Medical Journal*, 50 (Oct. 1926), 342–45.

Rayack, Elton. *Professional Power and American Medicine: The Economics of the AMA*. New York: World Publ. Co., 1967.

Reader, W. J. *Professional Men (The Rise of the Professional Classes in Nineteenth-Century England)*. London: Weidenfeld and Nicolson, 1966.

Real, Michael R. *Mass-Mediated Culture*. Englewood Cliffs, N.J.: Prentice-Hall, Inc., 1977.

Restak, Richard M. *Pre-meditated Man: Bioethics and the Control of Future Human Life*. New York: Penguin Books, 1973.

Ribicoff, Abraham. *The American Health Machine*. New York: Saturday Review Press, 1972.

Robinson, G. Canby., M.D. *The Patient as a Person*. New York: The Commonwealth Fund, 1939.

Rogoff, Natalie. "The Decision to Study Medicine," in Robert K. Merton, George G. Reader, M.D., and Patricia Kendall, eds. *The Student Physician: Introductory Studies in the Sociology of Medical Education*. Cambridge, Mass.: Harvard Univ. Press, 1957.

Rollins, Peter C. "Film and American Studies: Questions, Activities, Guides." *AQ*, XXVI, 3 (Aug. 1974), 245–65.

Rorty, James. *American Medicine Mobilizes*. New York: W. W. Norton, 1939.

Rosenberg, Charles E. *The Care of Strangers: The Rise of America's Hospital System*. New York: Basic Books, Inc., 1987.

———. *The Cholera Years*. Chicago: Univ. of Chicago Press, 1962.

———. "The Therapeutic Revolution: Medicine, Meaning, and Social Change in 19th-Century America," in Judith Walzer Leavitt and Ronald L. Numbers, eds., *Sickness and Health in America*, 2nd ed., rev. Madison: Univ. of Wisconsin Press, 1985, pp. 39–52.

Rosengren, Karl E., Lawrence A. Wenner, and Philip Palmgreen, eds. *Media Gratifications Research: Current Perspectives*. London: Sage, 1985.

Rothfield, Michael B. "Sensible Surgery for Swelling Medical Costs." *Fortune*, LXXXVII, 4 (April 1973), 110ff.

Schramm, Wilbur. "The Effects of Mass Communications: A Review." *Journalism Quarterly*, XXVI, 4 (Dec. 1949), 397–409.

———., ed. *Mass Communications*, 2nd ed. Urbana: Univ. of Illinois Press, 1960.

———. "The Nature of Communication Between Humans," in Wilbur Schramm and Donald Roberts, eds., *The Process and Effects of Mass Communications*. Champaign: Univ. of Illinois Press, 1971.

Schwartz, Harry. *The Case for American Medicine*. New York: D. McKay, 1972.

Scott, Ronald Bodley. "The Doctor in Contemporary Literature." *The Lancet*, 269 (Aug. 13, 1955), 341–43.

Settel, Irving and William Lass. *A Pictorial History of Television*. New York: Grosset & Dunlap. 1969.

Shafer, Henry Burnell. *The American Medical Profession 1783–1850. Columbia University Studies in History, Economics and Public Law, no. 417*. New York: Columbia Univ. Press, 1936.

Shorter, Edward. *Bedside Manners: The Troubled History of Doctors and Patients*. New York: Simon & Schuster, 1987.

Shryock, Richard Harrison. *The Development of Modern Medicine*. New York: Alfred A. Knopf, 1947.

———. *Medicine and Society in America 1660–1860*. New York: New York Univ. Press, 1960.

———. *Medicine in America: Historical Essays*. Baltimore: Johns Hopkins Press, 1961.

———. "Public Relations of the Medical Profession in Great Britain and the United States: 1600–1870." *Annals of Medical History*, new series, II (1930), 308–39.

Sigerist, Henry E. *American Medicine*. New York: W. W. Norton, 1934.

Sklar, Robert. *Movie-Made America: A Social History of American Movies*. New York: Random House, 1975.

Slaughter, Frank G. "Elements of Successful Novel Writing." *The Writer*, 85, 4 (April 1972), 17–19.

———. "When Scalpel Sharpens Pen." *The Writer*, 81, 7 (July 1968), 15–18.

Smith, Henry Nash. "Can 'American Studies' Develop a Method?" in Joseph J. Kwiat and Mary C. Turpie, eds., *Studies in American Culture*. Minneapolis: Univ. of Minnesota Press, 1960, pp. 3–15.

———. *Virgin Land*. Cambridge, Mass.: Harvard Univ. Press, 1950.

Spears, Jack. "The Doctor on the Screen." *Films in Review*, 6 (1955), 436–44.

Spivak, John L. *The Medical Trust Unmasked*. New York: Louis S. Siegfried, 1929.

Sprigge, S. Squire. *Physic and Fiction*. London: Hodder and Stoughton, 1921.

Starr, Paul. *The Social Transformation of American Medicine*. New York: Basic Books, Inc., 1982.

Stenn, Frederick. *The Growth of Medicine*. Springfield, Ill.: Charles C. Thomas, 1967.

Stern, Bernhard J. *American Medical Practice in the Perspectives of a Century*. New York: Commonwealth Fund, 1945.

———. *Society and Medical Progress*. Princeton, N.J.: Princeton Univ. Press, 1941.

Stevens, Rosemary. *American Medicine and the Public Interest*. New Haven: Yale Univ. Press, 1971.

Strong, Henry. *The Machinations of the American Medical Association*. St. Louis: The National Druggist, 1909.

Stuit, Dewey D., Chairman, and others of a subcommittee. *Predicting Success in Professional Schools*. Washington, D.C.: American Council on Education, 1949.

Suczek, Barbara. "Chronic Medicare." *Society*, 10, 6 (Sept./ Oct. 1973), 40–49.

Sykes, Richard E. "American Studies and the Concept of Culture: A Theory and Method," in Robert Meredith, ed., *American Studies: Essays on Theory and Method*. Columbus, Ohio: Charles E. Merrill, 1968, 71–92.

Tate, Cecil F. *The Search For A Method in American Studies*. Minneapolis: Univ. of Minnesota Press, 1973.

Tebbel, John. *The Media in America*. New York: Thomas Y. Crowell, 1974.

"There's A Doctor in the House." *TV Guide*, 18 (April 18, 1970), 41–44.

Thomas, Lewis. *The Youngest Science: Notes of A Medicine Watcher*. New York: The Viking Press, 1983.

Toffler, Alvin. *Future Shock*. New York: Bantam Books, 1972.

Trautmann, Joanne, ed. *Healing Arts in Dialogue: Medicine and Literature*. Carbondale: Southern Illinois Univ. Press, 1981.

Tunley, Roul. *The American Health Scandal*. New York: Harper & Row, 1966.

Tushnet, Leonard, M.D. *The Medicine Men*. New York: Warner Paperback Library, 1972.

Visscher, Maurice B., M.D., ed. *Humanistic Perspectives in Medical Ethics*. Buffalo: Prometheus Books, 1972.

Vogel, Morris J. and Charles E. Rosenberg, eds. *The Therapeutic Revolution: Essays in the Social History of American Medicine*. Philadelphia: Univ. of Pennsylvania Press, 1979.

Vollmer, Howard M. and Donald L. Mills, eds. *Professionalization*. Englewood Cliffs, N.J.: Prentice-Hall, Inc., 1966.

Waples, Douglas, Bernard Berelson, and Franklyn R. Bradshaw. *What Reading Does to People*. Chicago: Univ. of Chicago Press, 1940.

Warner, John Harley. *The Therapeutic Perspective: Medical Practice, Knowledge and Professional Identity in America, 1820–1865*. Cambridge, Mass.: Harvard Univ. Press, 1986.

Weinstein, James. *The Corporate Ideal in the Liberal State: 1900–1918*. Boston: Beacon Press, 1969.

Weiss, Walter. "Effects of the Mass Media of Communication," in Gardner Lindsey and Elliot Aronson, eds. *The Handbook of Social Psychology*, 2nd ed. Reading, Mass.: Addison-Wesley Publ. Co., 1969, pp. 77–195.

Wertham, Fredric, M.D. "The Scientific Study of Mass Media Effects." *American Journal of Psychiatry*, 119 (Oct. 1962), 306–311.

White, David Manning. "Mass Communications Research: A View in Perspective," in Lewis Anthony Dexter and David Manning White, eds., *People, Society and Mass Communications*. New York: The Free Press, 1964, pp. 521–46.

Wiebe, Robert H. *The Search for Order*. New York: Hill and Wang, 1967.

Wilbanks, Evelyn Rivers. "The Doctor as Romantic Hero." *Journal of the American Medical Association*, 220 (April 3, 1972), 54–57.

———. "The Physician in the American Novel, 1870–1955." *Bulletin of Bibliography*, 22 (Sept./Dec., 1958), 164–68.

Williams, William Appleman. *Contours of American History*. Chicago: Quadrangle Books, 1966.

Winn, Marie. *The Plug-In Drug: Television, Children and the Family*. New York: The Viking Press, 1977.

Wise, Gene. *American Historical Explanations: A Strategy for Grounded Inquiry.* Homewood, Ill.: The Dorsey Press, 1973.

Young, Francis Brett. "The Doctor in Literature," in Hugh Walpole, ed., *Essays By Divers Hands* (The Transactions of the Royal Society of Literature of the United Kingdom), New Series, XV. London: Oxford Univ. Press, 1936.

Young, James Harvey. *The Medical Messiahs: A Social History of Health Quackery in Twentieth-Century America.* Princeton, N.J.: Princeton Univ. Press, 1967.

Index

43; and the multiform image, 121–35

"Medical Center" (television program), 131, 133

medical profession: achievements of the, 32; before 1850, 19–25; between 1850 and 1870, 25–28; bureaucratization of the, 31–32; as a calling, 81–82, 84–85, 95–96; and the development of a body of knowledge, 20–22, 25; disillusionment about the, 32–34; European influence on the, 20–21, 27, 28; evolution of the, 4, 19–34; exposes about the, 33–34; as a male domain, 75–86; professionalization of the, 11–15; resistance to change by the, 31; revitalization of the, 28–29; since 1920, 29–32; status of the, 29

medical schools, 22, 23–24

medical science: advances in, 14, 23, 28, 44; before 1850, 20–21, 23, 25; and empiricism, 21; and epidemics, 23; European influences on, 28; funding of, 29; public attitudes about, 25, 27–28, 110–11; and uncertainty, 14

medical sectarians and cultists, 22, 24–25

medical societies. *See* American Medical Association; voluntary associations

"Medical Story" (television program), 133

medical training: as an ordeal, 12–13; before 1850, 19–20, 21, 24; and competence, 15, 21–22, 24; and the confidence of doctors, 15; and the creation of medical schols, 22; and the development of a body of medical knowledge, 12–14, 25; European influences on, 20–21, 27, 28; and limitations of the profession, 14; quality of, 24; reform of, 30; and the revitalization of the profession, 29; and the socialization of doctors, 4, 12, 15, 16; as a theme in paperback novels, 127; in Thompson's

writings, 116–17; and women, 82–83

medicine. *See name of specific topic*

Melville, Herman, 48

men, dominance of, 75–86

Menke, Wayne G., 31

Merrick, Bobby (fictional character), 112–13

Merritt, Samuel G. (fictional character), 93–94, 94

ministers, doctors' relationships with, 56–59, 63, 64, 98. *See also* religion and medicine; *name of specific fictional character*

Mitchell, S. Weir, 48, 59–60, 65–74, 87, 98, 99, 101, 102. *See also name of specific fictional character*

A Mortal Antipathy (Holmes), 65

Mortimer, Dave (fictional character), 113

Morton Family (fictional characters), 68–70

Mosses From An Old Manse (Hawthorne), 49

Mulbridge, Rufus (fictional character), 76–79

multiform image, 121–35

mystery (air of), 17, 71, 72–73, 89, 89–90

myths: function/purpose of, 2–3. *See also name of specific myth or image*

National Advisory Commission on Health Manpower, 32

New Jersey, 22

New York, 22

New York Academy of Medicine, 26

norms, 36

North, Owen (fictional character), 70–73, 74, 111

Not As A Stranger (Thompson), 104, 115–19, 121

Nye, Ephraim (fictional character), 89–90

Oakland, Richard (fictional character), 90–91

O'Hara, John, 47, 93–94, 96

About the Author

RICHARD MALMSHEIMER is a mental health therapist at Chambersburg Hospital in Chambersburg, Pennsylvania. He holds a Ph.D. in American Studies and an M.S. in Counseling. He has published in *Modern Fiction Studies*.